THE COUNTY

Adam & Jen,

I hope you enjoy my crazy stories. I hope this *is* such good for over the years like my there are families in Bellisan.

Fondly, Jason

The County

Surviving the Killing Fields

Jason M. Stoane, MD

ISBN-13: 9781505387797
ISBN-10: 1505387795

TABLE OF CONTENTS

INTRODUCTION

THIS BOOK HAS been many years in the making and consists of my recollections of events that occurred during my years of medical training at Kings County Hospital (the County) and SUNY Downstate (State University of New York Health Science Center in Brooklyn, New York), from 1988 to 1997. I started out as a medical student, did my medical internship, and then completed a four-year radiology residency. These stories are taken from my memories, and I'm certain that many of the tales have been embellished or even made up due to the vagaries of recalled memories of events that occurred years ago. I have changed the names of most of the characters in the book, because I wish to avoid causing them any undue duress. This artifice will hopefully allow me to freely tell the stories as I recall them. I have also refreshed my memory by scouring the Internet to fact-check my recollections. Fortunately, the *New York Times* has a site filled with articles about Kings County Hospital. The web was very helpful in filling in many of the gaps of my memory. In addition, I was able to revisit the stories from beginning to end, even if they occurred over extended periods of time.

"Killing Fields" was what the surgical residents used to refer to the medical wards at the County in A Building. I'm not certain when it started, but the name stuck for a reason, and I suspect by the end of this memoir, you will have a better idea why I, too, chose this name.

Dr. Walter Reed made one of the most important contributions to modern medicine, by confirming his theory on the transmission of yellow fever by mosquitos in 1901. He and I have something in common: we both did our internships at Kings County Hospital in Brooklyn. However, he had the sense to only stay four months. I was there for nine years. A plaque celebrating his life and achievements is probably still hanging near the entrance in the quietest part of the building, a hidden brick rotunda in B Building. These stories will memorialize the time I spent there for my boys.

Some refer to the "good old days." However, training at the County in the 1980s and 1990s should not be remembered as such. The building was in disrepair, as were many of the people. HIV and AIDS were ravaging New York City, as was a crack epidemic and violence related to drugs and poverty.[1] Racial tensions were running high. Resources at the hospitals were not.

Some of the stories are difficult to recount. Some of the stories are difficult to listen to. Viewing those times retrospectively is disconcerting. If you find a particular story too difficult to swallow, I would encourage you to skip it and move on. Each story is unique; however, the common thread is the unique time during which they occurred. Although I cringe at some of the things I said and did, I don't regret that I was there. I feel confident I did my best to help all my patients in the best way I could given the circumstances. I chose to go to medical school and train in Brooklyn because I thought a "hands-on" education would be the best way to learn medicine. Now, with the benefit of twenty years of medical practice, I believe I made the right choice.

My goal was to finally write down the stories I have been telling for years at cocktail parties and on ski lifts to my friends and family. I want my boys to have an unofficial record of their dad's life. I also want to retell these stories so that as our society moves forward

---

1 Mireya Navarro, "Treating AIDS: One Hospital's Struggle," *New York Times*, November 11, 1991.

into the new world of Ebola, we can learn some lessons from the past. By writing these stories down, my experiences and patients will not be forgotten. Hopefully, future doctors and policy-makers will have the benefit of my experiences as they wade through new epidemics that will assault our medical establishments.

The stories do not follow chronological order because I do not remember them in order, and they span the time I spent in Brooklyn from 1988 to 1997. As a twenty-three-year-old medical student, intern, and finally a thirty-one-year-old resident, I spent nine years working there. Sometimes, I lament that I spent my twenties shackled to the County, but I certainly gained a lifetime's worth of memories and tales I can share.

ACKNOWLEDGEMENTS

FIRST AND FOREMOST, I would like to thank all my patients for allowing me to take care of them during my training. They did not seem to care that I was a doctor in training. I think they were glad I was there for them.

I would also like to acknowledge my former instructors and friends who guided me along the way and allowed me to develop my unique brand of medicine, making the images tell me the patient's stories and vice versa.

I think it is well known that I had tried and failed to write this book many times. It took being in the right frame of mind, having the creative mental space, and the support of those in my life, both at work and at home. I want to thank my partners at NWR for all of their trust and support they have given to me. So many of my friends and colleagues at MBI and St. Joe's have had a positive impact upon me over the years that has helped make this project a possibility. I also want to especially thank Larry for inspiring me to go beyond my comfort zone again.

The editors at Create Space were invaluable. Without Create Space this book may not have been finished. In an instant, my new friend Joe Pa made the back cover text exactly what I had envisioned.

I am grateful that my family has always been supportive of my endeavors, no matter where they have taken me. My wife Chi-Na has always been my biggest fan and supporter, and I cannot express how important she has been in my life. She has always encouraged me to express myself in all the crazy ways I have chosen. She is a wonderful mom and a fantastic companion. I couldn't have picked a better person to go through all the good times and difficult moments side by side.

I also want to thank my boys, Caden and Asher, who are my pride and joy. They inspire me all the time. They have overcome so many challenges already. I hope they will continue to experience and enjoy all sorts of adventures during their lives. I hope that when they read this book, it will give them some insight into their parent's lives and will inspire them to follow their passions, wherever they take them.

1

THE STAPLE GUN

O N MY FIRST day on the surgical side of urgent care of the ED (Emergency Department), my resident taught me how to stitch a wound using instrument ties, a simple way of tying stitches into knots using surgical instruments instead of using your hands. He showed me how to make the knots with a needle holder (forceps). You push the curved needle through the skin and grab the tip with the needle holder. You wrap the suture material around the tip of the needle holder and then pull tight. To make a square knot, you reverse the process and make the second half of the knot in the other direction. He stressed that with silk as suture material, you need four throws to keep each square knot tight. He let me finish suturing a patient who had fallen and lacerated his elbow. It only required five more stitches, but it took me half an hour to complete all the throws.

My resident left to check on a patient on the floor, and I was about to pick up the next chart, when several police officers entered the urgent care room and asked for all the patients to be removed. The officers were decked out in riot gear and many had shotguns at the ready. Two burly officers brought in a prisoner who had both his hands and his feet shackled. They sat him down on a chair in front of me. He wore an orange prison scrub top. His forearms were exposed and had numerous lacerations, too numerous to count. Many of them were deep enough that they would require stitches. They were oriented horizontally and were likely self-inflicted.

I introduced myself as a medical student to the patient. The officers sitting next to him smirked at me. One of them told me he had been a paramedic in the military and would help me if I needed it. I told him, in jest, to remind me that I need to do four throws for each knot.

The patient was a thin black man, about six feet three inches tall, and 180 pounds. He didn't acknowledge me in any way. He stared right through me as if I didn't exist. I did not have the courage to ask why they had to clear out the room for this patient, but I suspect the police were worried he had injured himself so he would be brought to the hospital, where he might attempt to escape. I felt intimidated by both the patient and the cops.

I put on a mask and my gloves and started to stitch up his wounds using my newfound skill at performing the instrument knot tie. I was going as quickly as I could, but I wanted to do it right. Beads of sweat built up on my forehead, and I felt incredibly warm and uncomfortable. The officers were trying to get under my skin and engage me in conversation, knowing I was trying to concentrate. I could tell they enjoyed the fact that I was a newbie. The prisoner sat in front of me, emotionless and not showing any sign of pain the entire time.

About an hour into the procedure, the officers were less jocular and mainly watched me stitch. The patient continued to stare right through me until he said, "That was only three."

"Huh?" I responded.

The cop to my right laughed and said, "That was only three throws on that last knot!"

Behind my mask, my face turned bright red. I had no idea he was paying attention. I thought he was in some sort of trance. I apologized, completed the knot, and moved on.

A few moments later, my resident burst into the room. "What the hell is going on here?" he yelled. "Where the hell are all the patients?"

I said, "The cops cleared out the room for this patient and I've been stitching him up."

The resident looked at the prisoner's forearms, looked at what I had accomplished, and went over to the cabinets. He pulled out a package and brought it over. He opened it and placed a staple gun in my hand. The resident grabbed my hand and started to force me to staple the wounds closed. *Ka-chunk, ka-chunk, ka-chunk.* The patient continued to stare right through me and didn't even flinch.

"You should be done with him in two minutes. Get the rest of the patients back in here now!" he yelled at everyone in the room.

I regripped the staple gun and continued to staple his wounds. When I ran out of staples, I grabbed another staple gun and completed the job. My patient didn't say another word. The cops were pretty quiet, too.

2

THE BOXER

I PARKED IN the dirt parking lot and approached the entrance while I rummaged through my backpack to find my ID. The officers at the door were ready to harass me, so I needed to be prepared. Of course they let the homeless guys walk past them without raising an eyebrow, but they needed to interrogate the white guy wearing scrubs coming to work at the County.

I walked past the ER, which was filled, and took a left to go to "The Box." The Box is the radiology residents' reading room. It probably used to be a closet. It is dark and filled with two large film alternators, computers and monitors, and a few chairs. There is a door from the main corridor between C and B Buildings that enters into a dark alcove in front of the reading room. Radiologists interpret the X-rays in the dark using the backlit alternators to help bring out the subtle changes between black and white.

A large police officer was standing outside the entrance door. *Not too unusual,* I thought. There were hospital security guards, New York City police, and prison guards near the ER often, so I didn't think too much of it—until I entered the alcove and the large officer followed me in. Inside the alcove, another police officer was already standing at the door. Immediately, I felt how small the alcove was. I was sandwiched between two larger officers who were decked out in their usual paraphernalia of bulletproof vests, utility belts, and holsters containing guns. It was a tight fit there. I followed the officer in front of me as we entered the reading room. Pauli was dictating a case into the Dictaphone.

The officer in front of me said to Pauli, "Time to go. Stand up!"

Pauli said, "Can I take my backpack? It has all my books and I'd like to study."

The cop looked at him incredulously. "Uh, you're not going to need those."

Pauli looked at me and said, "Call the chairman. I need a lawyer."

I nodded my head in acknowledgement, still completely unsure what was going on in front of me, staring at Pauli with my eyes and mouth wide open, unable to speak.

Pauli said to me, in his thick Brooklyn accent, "I got into a little scuffle with a patient last night. Toby (the CT technologist) got decked. He's got some rib fractures on the films. You should read them. Okay?"

Pauli had two bloody scratches on his left cheek. "I was assaulted by a patient's 'friend' last night. When they arrested her, she pressed charges against me."

Pauli stood up, and the officer handcuffed him and escorted him out of the reading room.

I immediately called the radiology department chairman's office and told his assistant, Gloria, what I knew. Although the chairman was not in yet, Gloria said she would dispatch one of the young attending radiologists to go to the police station to bail out Pauli.

I ran upstairs to the hospital administration offices next to Walter Reed's plaque. I asked to speak with the administrator and filled her in. She mumbled, "Doesn't sound good. White doctor assaulting black visitor. Tell Pauli and your chairman he's suspended pending further review. He should not return to work until we clear this up."

I was shocked. I hadn't even mentioned the race of Pauli—or the visitor, because I didn't even know. They were reasonable assumptions, given that most of the doctors were white and most of the patients were black, but pulling the race card and suspending Pauli without due process infuriated me.

I went back to The Box and was greeted by Toby. He wanted me to read his X-rays. He indeed had two cracked ribs (nondisplaced posterior rib fractures) on his right side. He filled me in on what had happened the previous night.

The patient was a six-foot-two twenty-seven-year-old woman who had gotten into a barroom brawl. She was injured in the melee, but her partner, who was also over six feet tall, was not. The patient had neck and abdominal pain and needed a computerized tomography (CT/CAT) scan with contrast (dye injected into the vein to illuminate the organs) to exclude any internal bleeding. The CT scanner was located on the third floor in B Building so the patient was transported there. Her friend went with her for moral support.

Toby positioned the patient onto the CT scanner. Then he called Pauli to come upstairs and inject the contrast (dye) into the patient's arm IV for the scan. Immediately after he finished injecting the medicine, the patient began to scream. She said, "You're killing me. What did you inject me with?" "My arm is on fire!"

Her friend had been sitting in the hallway. However, when she heard the cries, she burst into the CT scanning room. "You're killing her! Get away from her!" the patient's friend said. She towered over Pauli, who is short and stocky—only five feet seven and 175 pounds. He was an amateur boxer and very strong and fit. He worked out at Gold's Gym regularly and would occasionally come to work with a black eye after a sparring misadventure. I told him he should give up boxing, because his eyes, hands, and brains were his best assets. I thought he was crazy to risk his career as a radiologist by boxing.

Pauli was trying to get to the patient to check her IV and assess her vital signs, but her friend stood defiantly in his way. Pauli told her to get out of the room so he could take care of the patient. He thought she was likely drunk or on drugs. She wanted to fight Pauli.

The tech said, "Doc, it's not worth it!" He tried to get between the two of them. The patient's friend picked up the seven-foot-long wooden backboard on the stretcher and swung it at Pauli. The backboard is pretty hefty, but she was very strong and very angry. She struck Toby and Pauli, who both fell to the ground. Toby was hurt worse than Pauli. As Pauli was recovering and tried to stand up, she came over to him and clawed at his face. He was able to grab her wrists, and they began to wrestle. Toby got himself off the ground, ran to the phone, and called security.

Pauli and the patient's friend continued to wrestle. Toby came over to pry them apart. Eventually, the security officers came running up the three flights of stairs and separated the combatants. Security felt that this was a police matter and got the city cops involved.

Pauli said he was okay and needed to attend to the patient on the CT scanner. She had fallen asleep! Pauli checked her out, and Toby completed the scan.

Blood was streaming down Pauli's cheek. He had drops of blood on his scrub top. The cops placed the patient's friend under arrest. She claimed she had been injured in the pelvis and had vaginal bleeding. The cops wanted Pauli to press charges against her, and she wanted to press charges against Pauli. All three were brought to the emergency room for treatment, and Pauli's face was cleaned up. Toby was taken to get an X-ray of his ribs. They placed Pauli under "house arrest" at the hospital, to allow him to continue to work, and told him that when his shift was over they would arrest him and bring him to the precinct.

I called Pauli later that day. He was at home and wanted to go to sleep. He said the police had dropped the charges against him and he should be able to go back to work in a couple days. It would give him some time off to study.

The police came back to interview me because I had interpreted the X-rays of Toby's ribs. They told me they planned on going forward with the prosecution against the patient's friend. Apparently, she had a long history of assault and battery and they wanted to put her in jail. They knew she was saying Pauli assaulted her in order to get the charges against her dropped.

3

Violating the Sabbath

A FEW OF the residents in my radiology program were Orthodox Jews. One Friday evening, I had just finished rounding on my patients on the wards, and headed to the bathroom in our call room (a suite where the residents could meet, study, and sleep if there was time). We were fortunate we had just become the beneficiaries of a remodeling and got a large break room with a kitchenette and a bedroom with an attached bathroom. Marty, the senior resident that week, was settling in for the night shift, sitting at the desk studying. The senior resident is available to perform all the ultrasound exams and invasive procedures at night. Marty was also Orthodox Jewish.

He saw I was headed toward the bathroom and he said to me, "Although I'm not really supposed to say this, could you remember to leave the light on in the bathroom? It's the Sabbath."

Although I am Jewish, I'm not up on all the rules and regulations of the Sabbath, but I know that observant Jews are not supposed to do any work on the Sabbath. I assumed that God grants special dispensation for physicians and others who are forced to work on the Sabbath. However, I figured that turning on the light in the bathroom was not allowed. In the bathroom, he had his toothbrush all ready with toothpaste on it, laid out on a paper towel. A cup of water was next to the paper towel.

I thought it was amusing that he could take call, do procedures, interpret studies, and render advice, but not turn on the light. I went to the bathroom, flushed the toilet, and washed my hands. I grabbed a paper towel and as I was leaving the bathroom, I automatically shut off the light. Before the door closed, Marty cleared his throat, loudly, with purpose.

I stopped in my tracks and exclaimed, "Jesus Christ!" I shook my head at myself, opened the bathroom door, and turned the light back on.

4

PACEMAKER

"Jas," MY MOM said slowly, "your Grandpa Bob has had a serious stroke. I'm not certain what to do."

"Mom, I'll make some calls and see what I can find out. I'll get back to you as soon as I know anything."

My grandfather Bob, my mother's father, had been in the hospital for the past week, recovering from a bout of congestive heart failure. He had recovered nicely and was supposed to be released that day. He had his first heart attack at sixty-two, and had received a pacemaker shortly thereafter, but it hadn't slowed him down much. After a few small heart attacks, he eventually underwent bypass surgery. He did very well after the surgery and had walked two miles every day for exercise religiously.

He retired to Florida and lived a happy existence with my grandmother Helen. Helen had bright orange hair and bright blue eyes. She was only about four feet eight inches tall. She was hilarious and could quote philosophy from Judge Wapner's recent shows perfectly. However, she knew very little about politics, news, or sports. She had lived in New York City her entire life until they moved to Florida, and she never had a driver's license. In fact, she had no solid identification, not even a credit card, though she did keep her Social Security card in her wallet with a stash of ones and coins. She was the "Sunshine Lady" for her condominium and sent out cards for birthdays.

Bob took care of all the important details of their lives. He paid the bills, prepared their taxes, and got things fixed when they were broken. Bob also chauffeured Helen and their friends. Helen had lived in NYC most of her life and had never learned to drive. Helen cooked the meals, Bob did the dishes.

I really enjoyed being around them. When I was young, they lived in Brooklyn's Flatbush Avenue area. I would visit them and go to Mets games with Grandpa Bob, even though he was a lifelong Yankees fan. We went to the Mets games because I liked them better, a huge sacrifice on his part.

Grandma Helen, with her silliness, always made me laugh. They had a large swimming pool behind their apartment building in Brooklyn, and when I visited them when I was a preteen in the summer, I would swim and play there for hours. However, Helen would make me change my swimsuit every half hour so I wouldn't catch pneumonia.

After Bob retired and they moved to Florida, I would still spend my college spring breaks at their retirement condo complex to hang out with them. I could study, swim, and run as much as I wanted in between games of gin rummy and shuffleboard. I could also borrow my grandfather's car and visit my dad's parents on my way to visit friends, who were enjoying the more conventional college-student spring break on the strip in Fort Lauderdale.

I tracked down Bob's primary care physician, and he told me Bob had suffered a major stroke and couldn't talk or move the right side of his body. I did the calculations in my head and figured that between his heart and now a major stroke, it was probably the appropriate time for me to be by his side. In my entire career to date (from 1992 to 2014), I have never called in sick and missed a day of work. I have had to reshuffle shifts to accommodate all sorts of events and calamities over the years (the birth of my son, the adoption of my second son, the flu…). However, I figured that this was a critical moment for my family and I needed to miss work and be by his side. My obligation to my work would have to come second this time. I was aware that my mom needed my help in confronting the uncertainties of Bob's future and coordinating his care. I called the chief resident and told him I needed a day off to be with my grandfather. He said he would find coverage, but I would owe it back. I agreed and called the airlines.

I flew down to Ft. Lauderdale, like I had done many times before, and rented a car. I drove immediately to the hospital where my grandfather was a patient. It looked brand new in comparison with the County. My grandfather was in a private room, sleeping comfortably, and I didn't want to wake him. He looked okay at first glance, but then I turned on my doctor mode. The right corner of his mouth was asymmetric, drooping slightly. His right hand was curled in on itself. His breathing was labored.

ECG monitors hung from the wall. Oxygen was piped into the room and there were numerous electrical outlets next to his bed, which also had multiple buttons for adjustments to make the patient more comfortable. We had none of these creature comforts at the County. A TV was at the foot of his bed. There was a sink in the room, and he also had a private bathroom. A large reclining chair was positioned next to his bed for family members such as myself. None of my patients at the County had a room that remotely looked like this one, and this looked standard for this hospital.

I told his nurse I was an intern at another hospital and asked her if I could review his chart. She agreed to let me. It did not look good. I went down to the radiology department and reviewed his brain scans with the radiologist—also not good. My grandfather had suffered a major embolic stroke to his middle cerebral artery supplying the left side of his brain. All the brain tissue covered by that artery was dead. The loss of function would typically include his ability to speak and understand speech and all motor function on the right side of his body. I had taken care of patients who were in the same predicament while I was rotating through neurology, and it was painful to picture my grandfather that way.

He was eighty-two years old and had a weak heart. He would never be able to walk again and probably wouldn't be able to feed himself. He might need a feeding tube entering directly into the stomach (a PEG tube) to avoid pneumonia from food particles going down the wrong pipe into his lungs because he could no longer swallow correctly. He probably would never learn to speak again, and he might not be able to understand language again. He would need to wear a diaper. He would need to be in a nursing home because Helen would not be able to take care of him—he had always taken care of her. My head began to spin.

I went to Bob and Helen's condo, changed, and went for a run. It was hot and humid. I began to sweat like crazy because I wasn't used to the humidity. I needed to clear my head and make some decisions. I jumped in the pool to cool off and swam some laps. We needed to figure out what Bob would want to do, even though he could not communicate with us. I needed to talk with Helen as soon as possible to figure out how aggressive we were going to be. Would Bob want to continue living like this?

I got back to the hospital a couple hours later. A pulmonologist was preparing to do a thoracentesis, a procedure to drain the fluid around the lung by sticking a needle into Bob's chest. He had my grandfather's side prepped and draped and was ready to insert a needle into his chest. I burst into the room and demanded that he stop. I asked him why he was doing this and from whom he got consent. He told me my grandfather had heart failure and had fluid on his lungs. He was going to take the fluid off so he could breathe better.

I told him my grandfather had bigger problems than his breathing at this time and I did not want anyone torturing him. I told him we could treat his fluid overload with medications and he did not need an invasive procedure. The pulmonologist said Bob's family physician had requested the consultation and he was just doing his job. I told him we did not need his services at that time and I would talk with Bob's family doctor right away.

I went back to the condo and had a heart-to-heart with my grandmother. I told her what I thought was going to happen to Bob and that we needed to decide how aggressive we were going to be with his treatment. My mom arrived and joined the conversation. We decided Bob would not want to continue living like this and we would take a conservative approach to his care.

I went back to the hospital to be with Bob. In his confused state, he had tried to get out of bed and fallen flat on his face, and now had a big bruise on his forehead. He was agitated and fighting with the nurses. His speech was unintelligible. It seemed as if he wanted to go to the bathroom, but the nurses were explaining to him, appropriately so, that he had a catheter in his penis and a diaper on, so he could relieve himself at will. He did not understand. The nurses placed restraints on his arms and legs to protect him from trying to get out of bed and hurting himself.

When he saw me, he recognized me and began to calm down. He shrugged his shoulders. I asked him how he felt and he shrugged his shoulders again. I told him what had happened to him, explaining that he had had a stroke. He shrugged.

I sat by his bed for the next eight hours. He would intermittently go to sleep and wake up and seemingly watch TV. I wasn't certain he understood any of it. After *The Tonight Show*, he fell asleep and his breathing became labored. He would stop breathing for long periods of time and I could watch his heart rate slow down. His heart would stop for a few moments and I thought he had died, but his pacemaker would kick in and start his heart again. He would wake up after these events for a moment, look at the TV, look at me, and then fall asleep again. This cycle repeated itself many times. At about 4:00 a.m., I couldn't take it anymore, figuring that his damn pacemaker was not going to let him die peacefully. I left the room, went into the waiting room down the hallway, and curled up on a couch. I had fallen asleep for about half an hour when a nurse came and woke me up. She said my grandfather had died a few moments before. I walked back down the hallway to his room and looked at him. He looked very peaceful. The heart monitor that had been torturing me had been turned off. I sat next to him for a long time, remembering all the good times we had spent together. I held his hand until it became cool. The nurse left me alone for a while. She came back in and asked me if she should call anyone. I thanked her for all she had done for us and went back to my grandparents' condo. I called my mom and she let everyone know. I picked up Helen and drove her back to the hospital to say good-bye to her husband of sixty years. I had no idea how she was going to take care of herself, but I knew she would be all right. My mom would make certain of it.

I spoke at his funeral and said he was the best grandfather a boy could ever ask for. He really was.

I flew back to New York a few hours after his funeral so I wouldn't miss my next shift at the County.

5

SKIPPING ROCKS

IF AN INTERN is not efficient in diagnosing and treating their patients, their patient workload will grow with every call. Not only is it incumbent upon interns to treat their patients, but oftentimes, they need to figure out whether the patient can be discharged. Because many of the interns at Kings County Hospital are foreign medical graduates (FMGs) and English may not be their native language, it is not unusual for interns to struggle. They struggle not only with the language, but with all the usual problems of being new. Of course, many of the patients don't speak English either. Many of the patients who use Kings County Hospital are Haitians and do not speak English, compounding the problems for the interns.

The interns all start July 1. (You never want to be a patient in July or August at a teaching hospital, when these newbie FMGs are trying to learn English, their way around the hospital, and medicine.) Interns start each month by inheriting the previous intern's patients. Generally, interns will inherit between eight and twelve patients. If they accumulate new patients during the month without being able to discharge any, they will create a mammoth service by the end of the month. Having a service of more than fifteen patients is difficult—twenty patients is nearly impossible.

The biggest service I ever saw was Eddy McDougle's. He was the first intern I was assigned to assist when I was a medical student, and though it sounds like he would be a red-haired Irish guy, he was from somewhere in the Middle East. He had a thick accent that made him difficult to understand and didn't have a clue about how to discharge a patient. Every four days he was on call and collected more patients. It was like Hotel California. He would admit them, discuss them on rounds, and try to do the assigned chores, but would rarely discharge any of his patients.

Since Eddy didn't understand the system, he was thwarted at every turn. It takes months to learn the in's and out's of the County. For example, to get a study like a CT scan approved by Radiology, you needed to come up with a really good reason to get the study done in an expeditious manner. You had to be willing to fight the system to get things done for your patients. This required time, persistence, and an excellent grasp of the English language. In the beginning, Eddy didn't have much of any of these qualities.

My nickname became Skippy. I earned this nickname as an intern. It refers to my ability to obtain "skips" in the rotation for interns on call. Every day there were four interns on call for the internal medicine service—two for each team. Every patient who gets admitted from the ER gets placed into "the book," which is a notebook with a rotation of the interns who are on call that day. The rotation goes from intern A to B to C and then to D, unless one of the interns has earned a skip. A skip in the rotation means one less patient to take care of. Generally, an intern will receive three to four new patients every fourth day, every time they are on call. A skip in the rotation can be earned two different ways. The first way to get a skip was to obtain an autopsy or small tissue sample, biopsy on a patient who died on your service (under your care). They offered this incentive to the interns and residents to help obtain material for the pathology residency program. However, getting family members to consent to an autopsy was difficult in the best of circumstances. First, there was the language barrier. Second, there were cultural barriers. For example, Haitians were very much opposed to doing autopsies based on spiritual grounds (because many practiced voodoo). However, some could be convinced to allow a biopsy. Third, many of our patients did not have relatives or family members whom we were aware of and could contact in the event that our patient died. Very few interns were successful at obtaining these skips. Too much time and effort.

The second way to get a skip was to discharge a "Rock." A "Rock" is a patient who has stayed in the hospital on the active inpatient medical service for more than sixty days. There are always about five rocks on the medical service at all times out of the hundreds of patients on the service. Although there are many reasons for a patient to turn into a Rock, the most common reason is that they don't have an address or place to be discharged to.

A patient is non-dischargeable if they do not have a local place to go or family who will take responsibility for them. When a patient is admitted to the hospital, a social worker will evaluate the patient's home life to see if the patient can be discharged. However, if the patient does not have a home to go to, the social worker would try to figure out an appropriate place for the patient to go.

However, if, after an investigation, there is no reasonable place for the patient to go, the social worker may give up. At the County, there were only two social workers on staff for the entire thousand-bed hospital. Many of the patients were homeless and destitute. Some came directly from JFK after flying in from the Caribbean (mostly Haiti) to get treated for TB or AIDS.

Haitians had their own unique cultural view on HIV/AIDS. Unfortunately, they were concerned that having someone in the home with HIV/AIDS would put the rest of the household at risk, so, if a son or daughter contracted HIV/AIDS—which was epidemic there—the family would kick the stricken member out. Some families would buy the sick member a plane ticket to New York, who would end up in the Kings County ER.

For example, at nursing station A72 (7th floor of A Building), my first Rock, Mr. Henri, had been treated for tuberculosis (TB) for five months and seemed to be otherwise healthy, although he was also HIV positive. He wandered around the wards in his hospital pajamas. He did not speak any English. He was one of those patients who had arrived at the County straight from JFK International Airport. He was Haitian and only spoke Haitian Creole. He was twenty-eight years old. I inherited him from the previous team and wanted to discharge him. However, because he did not have an address, he was deemed a rock and non-dischargeable. I decided to take on the challenge. I looked at the social worker's notes and found that his family in Haiti was afraid they would get AIDS from him and refused to take him back. He was in the United States without any family, and no one wanted him.

Fortunately, I'm pretty good at getting my point across in other languages. I spent a year as an exchange student in Belgium, which has three national languages: Flemish, French, and German. Melle is a small town outside of Ghent, in Flanders, where the main language is Flemish, a dialect of Dutch. After about three weeks, I was so lonely and stuck in my own thoughts that I was determined to become fluent in Flemish at all costs and refused to speak English. I learned to figure out the context of conversations by reading faces and gestures, and listening to the few words I could translate. After six weeks, I was functional in most situations, except on the telephone.

Haitian Creole has many French words, and I was able to communicate fairly well with my patients and their families.

I was able to strike up a conversation with Mr. Henri using French and the limited Haitian Creole I had picked up. I conveyed to him that he needed to get out of this place, as the hospital was the absolutely worst place for someone with a compromised immune system to be. The infections he could catch here were much worse than the ones he could catch anywhere else. I tried to convince him every time I saw him that he should just leave. He told me the other doctors wanted him to stay because he had TB. I told him his TB was under control and if he continued to take his medications, he would be fine. I told him he should go out and enjoy his life, not stay imprisoned at the County.

A few days later there were several important-looking people at the A72 nursing station. They were all dressed well. The nurse said they were looking for me. I introduced myself. One told me they were from administration and that another was Mr. Henri's father. The father wore a brown suit and black tie. He had a brown fedora in his hand. He looked like a successful businessman. They wanted to know why I was threatening his son.

I told them Mr. Henri had misunderstood my poor attempt to speak Creole. I had told him he didn't need to be treated in the hospital any longer and it was dangerous for him to stay. I looked his father squarely in the eyes and said, "The only reason he is still here, in harm's way, is because his family abandoned him."

His father looked at me hard and said in Caribbean-tinged English that the only reason he had not picked up his son was that he did not think he could get the care he needed in Haiti. In particular, he could not get the medications his son required. He would gladly take his son back home to Haiti if he could get the medications.

I promised him that for as long as he was alive, I would write the prescriptions for his son. The father could have someone fill the prescriptions here in New York and send the medications to Haiti. He seemed satisfied with this solution.

Every three months for the next two years, I received a letter from Mr. Henri's father asking for the prescriptions. I fulfilled my promise. Later, I received another letter from him thanking me for all I had done for his son, but he no longer needed the prescriptions because his son had passed away from complications from AIDS.

Another Rock I discharged was a patient I had inherited from the previous intern. She was a markedly overweight fifty-five-year-old who kept getting admitted to the hospital for shortness of breath and fatigue. She had been in the hospital for six weeks and the previous team had decided to keep her in the hospital, because she kept calling 911 when she felt short of breath. When I picked her up as a patient, she didn't seem sick at all. I reviewed her lab results and went over her imaging exams with the radiologists. She didn't have pneumonia, and, based on her recent CT scan, she didn't have chronic obstructive pulmonary disease (COPD).

It seemed to us her problem was she was overweight and probably had sleep apnea. My attending physician (supervisor) agreed with me that if I could find her an inpatient facility that would treat her obesity, I could discharge her. I called Weight Watchers in Manhattan, and they surprisingly had an inpatient facility and would accept my patient! The only catch was they wanted me to prove that she had sleep apnea. They wanted me to obtain blood from her artery (instead of the usual veins) with her breathing oxygen, and then one minute later without breathing oxygen.

This was a monumental task on the routine nursing station at the County, because the blood gas lab was in the Pathology Building down five flights of stairs, one building over and down two more flights of stairs. The blood had to be evaluated immediately, because the oxygen values would change and invalidate the test. I figured I had about 5 minutes if we put the blood into a cup filled with ice. I would have to place a needle into her radial artery in her wrist, extract the blood, have my medical student keep the needle in place, and run the sample to the lab. Then, repeat it again after we turned off the patient's oxygen supply.

We accomplished the task and the results came back affirmative. The patient was thrilled to find a potential solution to her long-standing problem. Another Rock discharged and a skip for me.

6

THE PATIENT I ALMOST
HAD TO MARRY

"N O WAY AM I taking care of her. She's dead!" I shouted at my
resident. He explained to me that I had no choice and it
would be easy. I objected vociferously.

"I'm a doctor and I take care of live patients. She's brain-dead
and needs a pathologist!" I said sardonically.

My patient, Ms. Toussaint, was a nineteen-year-old Haitian
immigrant in the United States illegally and staying with her family. She had lived here for about two years before she was caught in
her building when a fire broke out. She was not burned, but her
lungs were severely injured due to smoke inhalation. Tubes were
placed for her to breathe and receive nutrition and she was brought
into the intensive care unit (ICU). Her family wanted everything
done for her even though her condition was dire. Her brain had
gone for too long without getting enough oxygen from her damaged lungs, and she was brain-dead. Her body looked healthy, but
she would never regain consciousness. Her family members visited
her in the beginning, but when the social worker started to make

inquiries as to her legal status and payments for her care, the family stopped coming by.

A more permanent feeding tube was placed directly into the stomach through the skin, and a surgical procedure (inserting a tracheostomy tube) was done to give her a more stable long-term breathing solution. Even though she was brain-dead, she received the same care as any other patient. Ultimately, she was discharged from the ICU and placed on A51, one of the acute-care nursing wards. The nurses would shift her position every few hours so she would avoid getting decubitus ulcers. She was fed through her PEG tube, and she received oxygen and ventilator support through her tracheostomy tube. When she got pneumonia, the interns would prescribe antibiotics and she would get chest X-rays. If her tubes malfunctioned, specialists were consulted to fix or replace them. We were required to draw blood on her and do routine labs once a week.

I picked her up as a patient two years after she had been admitted. I was incensed that resources were being used for a brain-dead patient with no hope of recovery. I was told I was to round on her and write daily notes, as was required for every patient. If she had a fever, I was to evaluate and treat her like any other patient; find the source of the fever and treat it with the appropriate antibiotics.

I argued with my resident and refused to take care of her. He initially argued with me and then took a different approach.

"Come on, Jason; she'll be your easiest patient," he said. "Think about how much your medical students could learn taking care of her."

I was exasperated and demoralized. I wasn't going to dump this dead girl on my medical students like the hospital dumped her on me, but maybe they could learn a few things from taking care of her. I could let them be a little more involved than I normally would because there was no downside if they screwed up.

They could practice how to replace a tracheostomy tube, which would be riskier in a live patient.

Although I agreed to take her, I was not going to keep her. I was going to discharge her and get a skip. Watch me!

The first thing I did was run upstairs to talk to one of the social workers. Only two worked full-time in this thousand-bed hospital. Sounds ludicrous, but it was true. He scoffed at me when I told him I planned to discharge her.

"We tried," he told me. "Almost got it done, but when the emergency funds ran out, no one would take her."

She needed to be accepted by a "vegetable garden" (slang for a long-term care facility for patients in persistent vegetative states), equipped to take care of patients on ventilators and most can also take care of patients with feeding tubes. However, since she was not a citizen, no facility was going to accept her, because they were not going to get paid for her care. Even though taking care of her at an inpatient hospital, where she occupied a precious bed, cost many times more, the County could not move her.

"So," I said, "it sounds like the main issue is money, and behind that issue is her lack of US citizenship."

"Yes," he replied.

"What do I have to do to get her a green card? Marry her?"

He looked at me, startled at first, and then he smiled. His face changed, like he had an idea. He said, "You know, there is a way to get her citizenship if you really want to try."

"Tell me!" I said anxiously.

"Well, if you were to write a letter stating she would be unable to get the level of care she needs in Haiti, we could apply for a medical dispensation. Might work."

I agreed and wrote the letter. Needless to say, the wheels of immigration bureaucracy moved slowly.

During the two months I took care of her, I noticed several patterns. Her biliary enzymes would become elevated for no apparent reason. We would change her feeding tubes and the enzymes would normalize. She would get aspiration pneumonia about once a month and high fevers spiked. She responded well to standard antibiotics. She constantly had a urinary tract infection because of her Foley catheter. I instructed the staff to leave it out and use diapers, and she usually cleared up her infection with one dose of Cipro (Ciprofloxicin, an antibiotic).

My medical students learned to do many minor procedures on her as the need arose. I did eventually get her transferred to a lower level of care, where we only had to write notes on her three days a week and only ran blood work once every two weeks, or as necessary.

Every so often over the course of the next four years, I would receive paperwork about her citizenship request that required my signature. I had almost forgotten about her until, one day, as I was approving requests for ultrasound exams, I recognized her name on the request. She was still on A51!

The request was for a gallbladder ultrasound to rule out acute cholecystitis and biliary obstruction. I was incensed. I picked up the phone and paged the intern whose name was scrawled at the bottom of the request. He answered in a thick Middle Eastern accent. I asked him if he had dropped off the request on Ms. Toussaint on A51. He said he had. I asked him how long he had had her as a patient. He said he had just picked her up this week. I asked him if he knew that she was dead.

He paused, and then said, "My resident told me to request the ultrasound."

My blood began to boil. The same arguments arose in my mind from five years before. *This is madness! Why are we wasting resources on someone who will never recover? Can't someone make the logical and reasonable decision? She is only twenty-four years old and will probably live to be a senior citizen, if we continue to take good care of her. Think of all the money that is being spent on her!*

I told him the surgeons would never operate on her. "She would count against their mortality numbers (death statistics)," I said sarcastically. I told him to try changing her diet. If that didn't work, I would approve the ultrasound for the end of the following week.

The end of the next week came and a patient transporter wheeled her down for her ultrasound, much to my chagrin.

I performed the ultrasound exam on her myself, all the while thinking how ludicrous it was. We had such limited resources at the County, and using those precious resources on a dead patient was ridiculous. She had small gallstones. Her gallbladder looked fine, and, by the way, she had no pain over the gallbladder during the examination (the most specific sign of cholecystitis during an ultrasound exam).

A few months later, I got an invitation to a going-away party. At first, I thought it was for me because I was getting ready to graduate from my residency. When I looked closer, I saw it was sent from the nurses on A51. Ms. Toussaint had received her citizenship and had been accepted at a long-term care facility—finally!

7

ROAD RASH

I WAS STARTING a new rotation, and we were meeting at 9:00 a.m. Meeting late meant there wouldn't be any parking near the hospital. I started looking for parking on the streets several blocks before I normally would. Slowly, I turned onto Kingston Avenue, a one-way street. Unfortunately, because I was preoccupied with finding a parking space, I didn't realize there were two oncoming cars driving very fast, a red Honda Civic and a blue Toyota Tercel. It seemed they were jockeying for position and driving aggressively. I had accidentally interrupted their battle by turning into the middle of the road.

The cars passed me on either side and converged in front of me. I was going slower than both cars and watched as they almost crashed into each other in front of me. The game of chicken ended when the car on the left backed off, but lost control and sideswiped two parked cars. The damage was greatest to the front end of the Honda, but it wasn't the kind of crash where it seemed likely that the driver would be hurt.

The Toyota made the light and turned left onto Winthrop Street, joining the traffic. He made the next light as well and drove out of view. I passed the crashed cars and stopped at the light. I looked in my rearview mirror, and, as if in a scene out of *The Terminator,* the Honda that crashed into the parked cars came back to life. The driver backed up quickly to disengage from the injured cars and came up menacingly close to the back of my car. I wanted to get out of there, but I was stopped at the light and the traffic on Winthrop was at a standstill. I could tell the driver of the Honda was furious with me. He seemed to be cursing angrily and it looked like spittle was hitting the windshield inside of his car. He drove his damaged car within inches of my bumper.

I knew my presence on the road had contributed to the accident, and if I had been paying more attention to my surroundings, I wouldn't have made the turn at that time. However, in my mind, both drivers of the other cars were being reckless—I was driving like a little old lady and accidentally got onto their speedway. I had remorse that I was a witness to an accident, though, and the poor people whose parked cars were damaged would never know what happened. But I would not be reporting it; I had bigger problems.

Both the driver of the Honda and I realized simultaneously that he had nothing to lose and he could crash into my car without really hurting his car any further. Fortunately, at that moment, the light turned green and I was able to make the turn. However, we stopped a few feet later behind cars waiting at the next light and he pulled up his car behind mine. I locked my doors as he continued to yell at me from his car. Then he moved his car up and touched my bumper. He put it in park and got out of his car, ran up to my window, and screamed at me in Creole. I didn't understand it all, but I got the point.

I was scared he might have a weapon, but quickly determined that if he had a gun, he would have already brandished it. He was dressed for work in decent clothes and he was not very tall, probably five feet nine inches. He was thin and probably weighed 140 pounds. It wasn't that I was a good fighter, but I surmised that if this escalated into a physical altercation, I probably had the advantage. However, I had learned quickly in martial arts that you wanted to avoid all physical altercations, because you never knew what your opponent had up their sleeves and the bottom line was that I would get hurt even if I won the fight.

I felt emboldened because I hadn't seen a weapon and he was not physically intimidating. I also liked that I was in my car. He started to pound on my window. In front of me, cars started to move as the light turned green. We both realized I had a chance to get away now that he was standing on the street and I was in my car about to go. He moved to stand in front of my car and continued to berate me.

Now I had a one-ton advantage, but I wasn't going to run him down. Cars started to honk their horns and I slowly moved forward. He continued his harangue. Feeling the adrenalin surge in my veins, I gunned the engine in neutral to scare him out of the way. Instead, he jumped onto the hood of my car. I was shocked and now I was scared. I continued to drive forward slowly, now with his face just six inches from mine on the other side of the windshield. He continued to scream at me, but now I screamed back at him and continued to drive forward. This dude was not going to let go! I decided the best course of action was to get rid of this lunatic as soon as possible. I sped up to about 15 mph, crossed the double yellow line in the middle of the road separating traffic going in opposite directions, and drove down the street with him on my windshield still yelling at me. The light turned green at the next intersection and I turned in front of two lanes of traffic. He began to slip off the hood as I turned. He grabbed onto my radio antenna, which gave way immediately at its base, and he fell onto the pavement.

Fortunately, I was not going very fast. However, at that moment, I had little regard for his well-being. I wanted to get away from there as quickly as I could. I drove around the corner and did something I never done before or since: I parked in the parking garage. I stopped the car. My heart was about to pop out of my chest. *Shit! What just happened? Damn! I'm going to be late!* I thought. I grabbed my white coat and my dad's doctor bag and ran into the medical center, putting the last ten minutes out of my mind.

8

IN THE LINE OF FIRE I

My cousin Alexis was graduating from high school. My younger sister, Danae, came into the city from Connecticut, and we joined my aunt and my other cousins, Cindia and Brendan, for a celebratory dinner in Brooklyn Heights at a swanky restaurant and then returned to my aunt's brownstone in Park Slope, Brooklyn. After dinner we drove back to her place in "The Slope" and I double-parked across from my aunt's brownstone on Carroll Street. My sister and I got out to give everyone hugs before returning to my apartment a few blocks away. A red Camaro passed me as I was getting out of the car and double-parked about one hundred feet past us on the left side of the street. As I was crossing in front of my car, I heard *pop, pop, pop.* It sounded like fireworks to me, but the next sound I heard was glass cracking. I looked to the right at my windshield and saw it had a bullet hole in it associated with a crooked crack. My sister had been outside on the passenger side of the car and I surmised that the bullet must have gone right between us! I looked back up the street and saw flashes from a gun, coming from the basement of the brownstone directly across from the Camaro. One shooter was in the Camaro and the other was in a garden apartment on the left hand side of the street. The gunfire continued for a few more moments, but my sister, my cousins, and my aunt were all oblivious to what was going on until I began barking orders.

I yelled at my cousins and aunt to get inside their house, and I ordered my sister to get into the car. She complied, and I jumped in the driver's seat and kept my head down as I sped away up Carroll Street in the direction of my apartment. I saw in my rearview mirror the rest of my family hustling into their brownstone.

I don't think I took a breath until we were a couple blocks away. We passed Fifth, Sixth and then Seventh Avenue before I felt we were safely away from the situation. It was a beautiful sunny evening, and lots of people were out enjoying the weather. It seemed normal already, but we had just been shot at, and nearly hit by a ricochet bullet. *What the hell just happened?* I thought. *I guess I don't have to drive fast anymore.* Weird that everything seemed so normal. I guess it really was normal.

9

IN THE LINE OF FIRE II

L IVING IN BROOKLYN with a car means you have to keep everything locked down. Exposed loose change is a definite no-no. If you want to keep your radio, you either have to install a removable radio, which you take with you, or a radio with a detachable faceplate that you remove every time you leave the car. If you want to keep your airbag, you need to use the Club—a device that crosses your steering wheel and locks in place. You should also install special locks for your trunk and a kill switch for the ignition. Alarms are pretty useless because they're always going off and are generally ignored.

The worst part of getting something stolen from your car was replacing your car window. To get into the car, the thief generally breaks one of the windows. I have an inherent distrust of all New York repair guys, so I have my car fixed at my trusty mechanic in Connecticut near where my parents live, about a hundred miles outside the city. Every time my car got broken into, I would bring it back to my mechanic in Portland, Connecticut. Portland is a small town of about 4,500 citizens, about as diametrically opposed to Brooklyn as it can get, in every way except for the brownstones. In fact, the brownstone used in many of the homes in New York was taken from the quarries in Portland.

My mechanic was always interested in the stories I brought back from the big city. He had gotten used to replacing glass for a number of reasons, but replacing the windshield after being struck by a bullet was definitely a first for him.

The second time I was shot at I was stopped at a light behind the County. It was the same light I had been stopped at when the madman jumped on my hood. It was 10:35 p.m., and I was coming in to work the night shift in The Box. All the X-rays from the hospital were processed next to The Box, and the large manila folders containing all of the patient's X-rays and scans (X-ray jackets) were brought into the room on carts for the radiology resident to read and from which to dictate reports. The room was the size of a large closet and contained two alternators—large devices where most of the films from the night shift would be hung before being reviewed in the morning again with an attending radiologist. There were also computer screens on a desk behind the resident's chair, which were connected to an imaging system at Downstate, across the street; it was an early version of what we now call PACS (Picture Archival Communication System). Our director was prescient about the future of radiology. He had also installed two digital fluoroscopy units—pretty amazing technology for a county hospital where resources were always scarce.

I had just spent a wonderful week biking in Utah with my parents. We went with a bike-tour company called Backroads and flew in and out of Las Vegas. It was my first time to Vegas, and I was overwhelmed by the lights and the sounds of the city. Back then, Sin City felt a little greasier than it does today. We took a bus to Brian Head, Utah, and stayed overnight at a hotel. I was glad to be out of Vegas. Brian Head had a population of about a hundred people, and seemed to me to be about as far away from Brooklyn as you could get.

The hotel was over nine thousand feet above sea level, and I could feel the extra effort it required to bring my bags up the stairs. The hotel was nestled in the trees on a remote mountain.

We rode through southeastern Utah for a week and visited Bryce and Zion National Parks. What a great break from the hustle and bustle of living in New York City.

After finishing the trip, we went back to Vegas for our flights back home. I arrived back on the east coast in Newark Airport in New Jersey and took a cab back to Brooklyn. I got in at 9:30 p.m. I had just enough time to go directly to work. I flew into New Jersey because I had a direct flight and so the chance of something going wrong was minimized. I didn't want to leave anyone hanging out to dry at work because of a missed connection.

I drove my usual route to get to the County. It didn't take long as there wasn't much traffic. I came to a stop at the light. A car stopped as well, next to me on my right. I heard a loud sound. I wasn't sure what it was or where the sound came from, but then I realized my driver-side front window had been hit with a shot and a spiderlike crack appeared. I had no idea who had shot at me, or why, but I knew it came from my right. Even though it was dark and difficult to see well, I looked at the driver of the car next to me, to see if he was the shooter, but he was hunched down in his seat, looking as scared as I was.

The light was still red, but I wasn't inclined to just sit around waiting to get shot at again. My comrade in the car next to me had the same idea, and we both hit the gas. Initially, I just wanted to get out of there, but in a few moments, I realized I was out of danger. I pulled into my usual spot in the parking lot. In a heartbeat, I went from scared to angry. Now, with my window shot out, I couldn't secure the car and it would be a target for thieves. A broken window is an invitation for the bad guys to check out the contents of a car with impunity. And again, I had to drive back to Connecticut to get my window fixed. *I don't have time for this!* I thought.

I took my radio with me, placed the Club on my steering wheel, grabbed my backpack, and marched up to the entrance to the hospital. A hospital security officer stopped and asked me something. I heard a loud noise from the street and cringed. It was only a backfire, but I was strung so tightly, I nearly dropped to the sidewalk.

The security officer approached me and asked me again, "Would you be willing to donate some money so we could get bulletproof vests?"

Are you kidding me? I thought. *I just got shot at and you guys need vests?*

10

ASIAN FLU

TOMMY WAS ONE of my best friends in my radiology residency. Tommy was first-generation Chinese and was dating a Jewish girl. This was a big deal for his family, particularly his father, who wanted Tommy to be with a Chinese woman. Tommy had invited me out a few times to meet his Asian friends, because, he said, I had "Yellow Fever." What he meant was that he thought I found Asian women attractive. The fact of the matter was that I dated many different women over the years and I think my main criteria were that they be gorgeous and smart, and could tolerate me. The last girl I had dated was Columbian. The previous one was from Ghana.

Tommy was covering the night shift one week when he asked me to come in early, at 5:00 a.m., to cover for him on Saturday morning so he could drive to Atlantic City. He was planning to "pop the question" to his girlfriend. I agreed, of course.

I woke up at 4:00 a.m. I had made some eggs, and I was sitting at my kitchen table and reading a new issue of the radiology journal I had subscribed to. I could barely focus my eyes. There was an article with a title something like "Os Odont"—something to do with the cervical spine, which they weren't sure was a birth defect or related to old trauma. Although I wasn't awake enough to fully understand, the article showed images of damage to the spinal cord if it went undiagnosed.

I drove my car to work so I could relieve Tommy from The Box early, so he could propose. I knew this was a big deal for him, mainly because his dad was going to explode when he heard about it.

I sat down and got myself ready for the shift. The first case was a cervical-spine X-ray series of a patient who had an odd looking second vertebra. The tip looked broken and was tilted backwards towards the spinal cord. *What the heck was the name of the syndrome I had just read about? Os Odont.* I grabbed a textbook and found it: "Os Odontoideum." Amazing coincidence! I don't believe in fate, but this was really weird. I called the ED doc and explained to him what the syndrome was and that he should have the neurosurgeons take a look at the patient. If I hadn't read that article while I was eating breakfast, I never would have known about this syndrome and would have missed the finding or misinterpreted the findings, and this patient might have gone on to injure her spinal cord. How random is that?

Ultimately, Tommy backed out of the engagement and, to the delight of his father, went on to marry a Chinese girl.

11

OVERDOSE

D R. HALLER CALLED me up and said, "We need to talk."
I wasn't sure what I had done wrong, but it didn't sound good.
I went down the hallway to his office. Dr. Haller was a famous pediatric radiologist. He had a caustic sense of humor, and was incredibly smart and a charismatic leader.[2]

When I entered his office he held up vials of fentanyl and Versed and asked me, "Do you know what these are?"

About the time I started my interventional radiology rotation was when we started to routinely use conscious sedation for virtually all our procedures. Interventional radiology is a relatively new field where radiologists use imaging in order to guide needles or catheters into patients. Many of these procedures are minimally invasive, but can still be quite painful. For example, we had started doing a new procedure called TIPS (transjugular intrahepatic portosystemic shunt).

TIPS procedures are done on patients with cirrhosis (liver failure generally from long-term alcoholism) who have severe portal hypertension (the blood couldn't get through the liver and began

---

2 Unfortunately, he died from pancreatic carcinoma at the age of sixty-two, shortly after I left Brooklyn.

to back up creating new routes around the liver). The first step is to put a needle into the patient's jugular vein using ultrasound guidance. Then, we place a wire through the needle down into the heart. Using dilators, we upsize the catheter to a very large working catheter, which I call a "cannon." We advance the cannon through the heart and then advance a smaller catheter through the cannon into the liver into the middle hepatic vein. At that point, we advance a scythe-like needle (called a Colapinto needle) into the middle hepatic vein and take swipes through the patient's liver, trying to find one of the portal veins. Often, it takes multiple attempts to get into the portal vein. Once we have access to the portal vein, we place a stent bridging the portal vein and the hepatic vein, bypassing the diseased liver.

TIPS procedures can take hours to accomplish and can be very painful. It's necessary for the patient to hold very still and be cooperative. Until recently, radiologists had not used medications to sedate patients. Notice, radiologists perform *procedures*, not *surgeries*. Although this may seem a merely semantic difference, most radiologists are squeamish about hurting patients. Traditionally, radiologists read chest X-rays and mammograms, but at the County, radiologists did that as well as TIPS procedures, and more.

"Sure!" I replied to Dr. Haller.

"Well, we found them in the call-room bed on Monday morning, right after your last shift."

I reached for the breast pocket of my scrubs. "Uh, yes. I pulled the meds for conscious sedation for the weekend patients."

"You shouldn't do that," he said. "Nuff said."

"Got it," I replied.

In retrospect, it was unconscionable that I would have these powerful and addictive medications on my person, but at the time it seemed not unreasonable. As residents, we ran the show after the attending radiologists went home in the evening. We would read all the X-rays, ultrasounds, CT scans, and MRIs; and the

ER doctors and surgeons would act on what we had to say. In the mornings, the scans and whatever X-rays could be found would be reviewed by an attending radiologist.

In addition, we residents would perform procedures on our own, without any supervision. One of the first things I would do, when I was working nights as a senior resident, was make up two angiogram trays. Gary, my former chief resident, had showed me how to make up sterile trays so I could perform an angiogram essentially unaided, with minimal assistance from the CT tech.

"Angios" were routinely performed on patients who had been stabbed or (more frequently) shot, and who might have a blast injury to the inside of a major blood vessel. When a bullet passes through the leg, for example, there is a concussive effect on the surrounding tissue. The bleeding generally comes from lacerated veins, tiny arteries, and the muscle and bone. Most of that bleeding can be stopped by compression. Large artery bleeding would need to be repaired either by surgery or by placing small amounts of sponge (gel foam) into the bleeder through a catheter. However, the larger concern comes if the bullet caused an injury to the inside of the artery by the "blast effect," which could cause a delayed occlusion of the artery and bigger problems. The trauma doctors needed this information ASAP and we would bring the patient directly to the angio suite.

Similar to coronary angiograms, a needle is inserted into the femoral artery in the groin. Then a wire is placed through the needle, take the needle out, leaving the wire, and then advance a plastic tube over the wire. Of course, we clean the groin and anesthetize the site, but it's still uncomfortable. Although the procedure is usually over in thirty minutes, we found that giving the patients some drugs usually made it go easier for both the patient and us. Since we didn't have a nurse at night or on the weekends, I would take fentanyl and Versed from the nursing cart and administer it to the patients as necessary to get them through the procedure.

Just for the record, I have never used drugs. I barely drink alcohol—I do it to be sociable, but I generally regret it the next morning. I have been described as a "cheap date." When I went to the Caribbean with friends, our boat pilot said I was the first person he had ever met who didn't drink when vacationing in the Caribbean. For me, drinking does nothing to enhance my sense of a good time. In fact, it usually makes me a little depressed and sleepy. It never dawned on me why hoarding drugs for performing procedures on patients was such a terrible idea, until—

"Doc, it's Jennifer, she's dead!"

Jennifer had come to Brooklyn to become an X-ray tech. She was super friendly, and she worked really hard. She was also very smart, having graduated from Cal Tech. Many of us recognized she had potential she was not tapping into. Being a tech is a good job, but Jennifer could have done much more. She applied and got into medical school at Downstate. She worked harder than anyone and seemed to really enjoy the rigors of the program. Over the years, we would see each other around the hospital, and she always seemed to have a smile on her face.

She made it through the first two years of med school and had started doing her clinical rotations. She seemed as if she had her life dialed in. Once, when she was on her "peeds" (pediatrics) rotation, she mentioned that she had always wanted to go to Africa and take care of the kids there.

She was found in the tiny, dingy operating room darkroom. The OR darkroom was located next to the entrance of the operating room. It is where X-rays that are taken in the OR can be developed and processed rapidly. Jen was found sprawled on the floor, lifeless. Drug paraphernalia was lying next to her body. She was in her scrubs. There were multiple glass vials on the ground containing fentanyl. Fentanyl is a very potent narcotic analgesic that is injected into the bloodstream and works in seconds. It's used for pain relief in simple procedures. It's an amazing drug, but it was becoming the drug of choice to abuse. I had heard that some doctors were abusing fentanyl around the country, but I was shocked that Jennifer of all people would OD!

Was it suicide? Was she stressed out? I asked myself.

I found out later that she may have been using drugs for some time to stay awake to study, and to relax and sleep when she needed to.[3]

3 Dave Kocieniewski, "Medical Student Found Dead, and a Painkiller Is Suspected," *New York Times*, November 7, 1995.

12

How I Met My Wife

"I've been looking all over for you. Could you just approve the CAT [CT] scan? My resident said I needed to get it done."

"Uh, I'm actually a little tied up right now. I have a catheter in this patient's carotid artery and we are about to shoot an angiogram. Could you step out of the room?"

I was scrubbed into the case. I was sterile: wearing a surgical mask and gown as well as a lead apron and vest underneath that. I was about to step out of the room as well so the tech could inject the contrast and turn on the X-rays to take pictures of the dye being pushed out of the catheter into the patient's carotid artery. He had been stabbed in the neck, and I was asked to evaluate the arteries for additional injuries. He had gauze on his wound, but it was soaked through with blood. At one point, the gauze fell off and the open wound was pumping out blood. I got some new gauze and applied pressure for a few minutes before I started the procedure. I taped it on with an adhesive, which seemed to stabilize the situation and stopped the bleeding enough so I could complete my procedure.

It is always nerve-racking when you have a catheter in the carotid artery. I've never gotten over the feeling that I might cause a stroke at any moment during the procedure. A clot can build up on the catheter or wire; I could accidentally inject some air…These thoughts go through my mind every time I advance a catheter into someone's carotid or, even worse, into the vertebral artery. A stroke in the posterior circulation, from the vertebral artery distribution, is often devastating.

Like a quarterback in the pocket trying to make a pass downfield before he gets crushed by the incoming blitzers, I have an internal clock ticking in my head for how long I have before I either need to flush the catheter to remove clots or move it out of harm's way. Once we hook up the catheter to the injector, it's "go time" and we need to inject the contrast, shoot the images, and clean the catheter. In other words, there's no time for chit-chat or to consult with an intern about a CT scan.

As I stepped out of the room and moved past her, I made certain my gloves and gown did not touch her in any way, to stay sterile so I could move back into the room immediately after the images were obtained. As I nodded to the tech and gave the patient last-minute instructions, the intern started to tell me she needed to get the scan approved and done that night. Her persistence was remarkable, as was her nearly perfect English. I looked at her badge and saw her name was China Kim. She was very pretty. She wore blue-gray scrubs with a T-shirt underneath. She was about five feet three inches tall and very thin, but you could see she worked out. Her arms were sinewy, and her cephalic veins were visible on her biceps. She carried herself regally. You could tell there was a lot of power in that small body. She was clearly Asian, but I wasn't certain whether she was Chinese or Korean. I spent a year abroad as an exchange student and pride myself on noticing little details that hint at a person's place of origin. I have an excellent ear for accents and can navigate several languages.

Last name, Kim. Must be Korean. She spoke English much too well to be an FMG and I suspected she was not an intern in internal medicine. Kings County Hospital has one of the largest residency programs for primary care in the country. Primary care includes internal medicine, pediatrics, family practice, and OB-GYN. One can enter different specialties after completing a three-year internal medicine residency (such as cardiology, gastroenterology, and hematology/oncology).

At the time, the highest-paying specialties were orthopedics, ophthalmology, and cardiac surgery. The lowest-paying specialties were internal medicine, family practice, and pediatrics. Although the majority of my classmates in medical school professed at the beginning of our first year to want to save the world and become family physicians, by the time we made our choices in our fourth year, most of us (me included) had opted for more lucrative specialties. At the County, virtually all of the interns in internal medicine were FMGs. Although she was Korean, a foreigner, she had a different look, more sophisticated than most of the residents. *She must be one of the new ER residents who was forced to rotate on the Killing Fields*, I thought. The County was starting a new ER residency and there were about twelve doctors who joined up. Even though they had done internships elsewhere, they were now obligated to do another one. Emergency medicine had only become an officially recognized specialty in 1979, but Kings County didn't start its program until after the Crown Heights riots in 1991. Until then, the ER at the County had an assortment of attending physicians taking care of acutely sick and injured patients. Very few of them were specifically trained in emergency medicine, like Dr. Kildare Clarke, who was a psychiatrist and, at one point, the highest-paid city employee.[4] Emergency residencies attract excellent candidates, partly because ER doctors earn decent money—usually better than internists, family docs, and pediatricians—and partly because of the popularity of the TV series *ER*, which began airing in 1994.

4 Josh Barbanel, "Doctor at Kings County Earned $259,679 for Year," *New York Times*, October 2, 1991.

I later found out that her name was Dr. Chi-Na Kim, and she indeed was Korean and a new ER resident. She was toiling in the Killing Fields this month, getting tortured by the County, like any sane doctor. She was sent on a suicide mission by her resident: at the County, to get their patients diagnosed and ultimately discharged from the hospital, most doctors need to get imaging studies done as well as consultations from specialists. Like many city institutions, the goal of virtually all the employees is to do as little as possible, get paid, and go home (or go to a second job) at the end of the day.

To get any high-tech imaging studies done, preauthorization was required, similar to that required by many insurance carriers today. The preauthorization was performed by the more senior residents, and for the most part, they also were trained by their forebears to do as little as possible so they could do other things—namely, study for the boards. The interns had to run the gauntlet to get their studies approved. Radiologists, if I do say so myself, are oftentimes the smartest doctors in the hospital—think Sheldon from *The Big Bang Theory*. To get a CT scan approved, interns have to present their rationale.

In defense of the system, and the individuals whom I just derided, there are very limited resources available and those resources need to be utilized as judiciously as possible. At the time, the County had only two CT scanners. Both were single-slice scanners (1970s technology), and each study took about thirty minutes from start to finish. During the day, one of the scanners was primarily utilized for image-guided procedures (mainly complex abscess drainages and needle biopsies). The County was a thousand-bed Level 1 Trauma Center. (For perspective, my current hospital in Bellingham, Washington, is a Level 3 Trauma Center with two hundred beds and two very fast CT scanners.) We often did not have transporters, and IVs (intravenous lines) were started by the radiology residents, who also hung the films.

Chi-Na was sent to get approval for her patient, a prisoner from Rikers Island, on whom she was told to get a CT scan of the brain with injected X-ray dye (contrast). I could tell from her tone of voice she didn't really think her patient needed the scan, and she was just getting her errands done. The request made of her was idiotic because the patient had already had an MRI (magnetic resonance imaging) the day before, which is a much better exam anyway. Kings County Hospital did not have an MRI at the time.

Magnetic resonance imaging is more sensitive and specific than CT scanning for most diagnoses of the nervous system. It was invented by Raymond Vahan Damadian in 1977 at SUNY Downstate, the building across the street from the County.[5] In order for a patient at the County to get an MRI, they needed to be transported by ambulance literally across the street.

As it turned out, I was reading MRIs this week. When Chi-Na showed me her request form, I recognized her patient's name and recalled that his MRI was normal. I remembered him because it was such a big deal to get him transferred across the street; he was a prison-ward patient, which required cutting through additional red tape to get him across the street. He also had no IV access, because he was an intravenous drug abuser, and I spent about half an hour trying to get IV access.

The first thing I did was ask her whether he really needed the exam. She hesitated—a key mistake. She then went on to say she needed to get it done so she could discharge him. I told her that to do any exam—especially one that required an injection of contrast, which was potentially fatal if he were to have an allergic reaction—she needed to give a reasonable rationale.

---

5 Damadian received the initial patents for MRI; however, he was snubbed by the Nobel Committee, which would later award the 2003 Nobel Prize for Medicine to two other researchers in the field of diagnostic imaging, Paul C. Lauterbur and Sir Peter Mansfield.

I felt bad for her, because she was clearly being tortured. I offered her some words of advice from my years of experience at the County.

"When you want to get a CT scan of the brain with contrast approved, there are a few key words that would be helpful," I told her. "For example, does your patient have an altered mental status? He is at Rikers Island, after all. He has AIDS. If you put AIDS and altered mental status together, it buys him a scan. Who knows...He could have meningitis."

She looked at me and said, "I cannot lie. I'll get down on my knees and beg, if it will help."

"Uh, this is going to be a long, difficult time for you here. I wasn't suggesting that you lie; I was just saying there are certain key phrases that could be effective in getting your exams approved. Anyway, if you can get him down here—knowing it would be next to impossible in the middle of the night—I'll stick him and get his scan done."

I signed the CT request form she had brought and she delivered it to the CT tech. Later that night, the prisoner was escorted into the CT suite by two large corrections officers. I saw him shuffling down the long corridor between A and B Buildings. Both his hands and his feet were shackled. They sat him down in the IV chair. Toby, the tech, called me, and I came to get his consent and place his IV. Knowing how hard it was going to be to place the IV, I decided to consent him for the injection of the contrast medication first.

I gave him my informed consent contrast spiel. "I am going to try and place an IV again. This dye is different than the MRI dye. This dye has a greater risk of allergic reactions. The risk of serious reaction is unpredictable and unpreventable. The risk of death is small."

He interrupted me at that point, waved his hand across his throat, and said he wanted to go back to bed. He got up and the officers escorted him back to the prison ward.

That's how I met my wife.

13

HOW I MET MY WIFE II

"**I**'D LIKE TO get an ultrasound of the gallbladder when you get a chance." Chi-Na had called me at 4:00 a.m. I was the senior radiology resident on call, and it was my responsibility to either do the exam or triage it to the morning. Many radiology residents would have punted it to the day shift.

"OK, if you bring her up right now, I can do it," I responded.

"Uhhhh, it's not that urgent," she hesitated.

"If you bring get her up here now, I can get it done and out of the way. You never know what is going to come in later. I'd rather get it done now."

"OK," she said a little surprised.

Chi-Na transported the patient herself and arrived at the ultrasound suite 15 minutes later.

The patient was a middle-aged, overweight, black woman with pain in the right upper quadrant of her belly. She had a southern accent that I had detected during our introductions. I always try to chit-chat with the patients while I am doing the exams in order to make them more comfortable. If they are relaxed, the patient is more likely to allow me to push as hard as I need to with the ultrasound probe, and not hate me in the end.

When I started medical school at Downstate (aka State University of New York Health Science Center at Brooklyn), we were given a document about the demographics of the population of Crown Heights at the time. One large population spike on the graph was from Georgia. Over the years, I had taken care of several of these patients, and found out that many of them came from one area, Randolph County, in south east Georgia.

As I started the exam, I said, "I bet you didn't know by my accent, but I'm a "southern boy". I said in my plain-Jane northeastern accent to the patient. "I was born in Nashville, Tennessee. (*I carefully said I was* **born** *in Nashville, because I only lived there for the first six weeks of my life before my parents moved the family back to New York and I have never been back since.*)

"I bet you are from Randolph County Georgia," I said.

She broke into a big a smile, even though I was pressing hard into her belly fat with the probe in order to see her gallbladder and bile ducts. She replied, "Why, yes, doctor. How did you know?"

"Bet you miss the sunshine," I said. It was January; dark and cold. We had just had a snowstorm last week in the city.

"Suuure do," she replied with a heavy southern drawl.

She seemed pretty happy thinking about Georgia and allowed me to perform the exam without complaint.

As I was finishing up, I told Chi-Na that I was about to finish a long week of call in a few hours. She asked me what I was planning on doing.

"I was thinking about heading to Connecticut to my parent's place and going skiing." "Want to come?"

She said, "I'd love to go skiing."

Before we wheeled the patient out of the ultrasound suite, she handed me her phone number. I said that I would call her after I woke up and I could swing by and pick her up. I love skiing and finding a girl who will go with me sounded awesome.

Later that day, I woke up more tired than when I went to sleep. I did not feel up to getting my gear ready and driving several hours to go skiing. But, I did want to get together with Chi-Na. I was in between girlfriends and she was smart as well as cute.

I called her up and we set up a lunch date in Park Slope. I picked her up at her apartment. She lived about 14 blocks away in a one bedroom apartment right next to the subway. It was the elevated part of the N train, and she lived on the second floor. The subway literally ran right next to her window. Fortunately, she was an intern and mostly slept at the hospital. Even when she was home sleeping, she was too tired to even notice the small earthquakes that shook her apartment every half hour.

It wasn't until much later when we were skiing in Colorado that Chi-Na confessed to me that she didn't know how to ski at the time of our first date. She claims she said, "I'd love to go skiing." Emphasis on the I'**d**, as in I **would** love to go skiing if I knew how. The way I heard it was that she **loved** skiing and wanted to go with me.

Her defense was that she claims I was also being dishonest. Being born in Tennessee does not qualify me as a "southern boy."

14

SLEEPLESS IN NEPAL

ALTHOUGH I HAD decided to go into radiology and had matched[6] to Downstate for my residency, I still had to complete a preliminary year. I could choose internal medicine, pediatrics, surgery, or transitional (hybrid) internships.

My father is a radiologist. He is very different from me. He is exceptionally smart, a member of Mensa, and very exacting about what he does. He's a mathematician or an engineer at heart. It takes him an hour to get ready to go biking because he needs to prepare everything: check the weather, get the right socks and shirt on for the weather, pump up the tires, and so forth. As for me, I like to figure things out as I go along. I am a firm believer in my ability to adapt to almost any situation. I have no problem getting on my bike and winging it. Because we are so different, I never imagined I would follow in my father's footsteps and become a radiologist. I certainly never thought I was as smart as he is.

After I lived in Belgium, I knew I could learn languages quickly, so I thought I would have a career in international relations or international politics. Even when I found myself in medical school,

6 The "Match" is the day that most US medical students find out which residency programs have chosen them. See http://www.nrmp.org/residency/

I gravitated toward the "doer" specialties. I admit freely that once I was exposed to ENT (ear, nose, and throat) surgery, I was smitten. As I went through medical school, I realized I loved the intellectual challenge of medicine as much as the "doing" challenges. I also found I was able to make the sacrifices necessary at all levels of my life to be successful.

I told my dad I was interested in becoming an ENT surgeon and he told me to talk to his friend, a local ENT physician in Middletown, Connecticut. He said it was hot and sexy in training, but in private practice, it could be quite boring and mundane—lots of time in the office seeing patients with allergies and ear infections. All the cool difficult surgeries were done at the "Meccas," the teaching hospitals. I could tell he was bored.

There were only four American grads out of eighty internal medicine doctors in training at Kings County Hospital: Marshawn, Reggie, Emmy, and I. All radiologists had to do a one-year internship of either internal medicine, surgery, pediatrics or a transitional (hybrid) internship prior to starting in radiology, but the fact that my parents owned my co-op in Park Slope and gave me a break on the rent, that my dad trained at SUNY Downstate and was also an attending radiologist at Downstate, that Lucy Frank Squire—the grand dame of radiology—spent her career there, that MRI was developed there, and that radiology seemed to run the whole hospital, all made me want to stay for radiology.

Staying for my year of internal medicine was considered sheer madness by my friends, but the city of New York was desperate for American graduates to stay in the program and offered a special scholarship to those American medical-school graduates who would be willing to work at the city's hospitals in primary care.

Marshawn grew up in Brooklyn and always hung out with the black medical students during class. He confided in me that his mother had died of AIDS a few years before. He was tough as nails. He had street smarts and nobody messed with him.

Reggie was a native New Yorker. He was about five years older than the rest of us. He struggled through medical school, but made it. He seemed to always be tired and have a five o'clock shadow.

Emmy was a Chinese immigrant. Though she had lived in New York for fifteen years, she still had a thick Chinese accent. She had hung out with the small group of Chinese students during medical school and I didn't get to know her well.

My three comrades had committed to the internal medicine program for three years. Even though I was only doing one year, the director still gave me the scholarship. I also negotiated one more condition for me to stay at the County: I wanted one month of elective leave when I could go to Nepal. Early on, however, the FMG residents learned of our extra stipend and were resentful, understandably.

Just prior to graduating medical school in April 1992, I decided to do an Outward Bound program in southeast Utah for an entire month. (I took out a student loan to pay for it!) It was an amazing month out in the La Salle Mountains backcountry, camping, rock climbing in Canyonlands National Park, and rafting down the San Juan River. It was quite a contrast from New York City living. We were away from cell phones, beepers, smog, and car alarms for a long time. And there was a lot of time for reflection—something I rarely did.

When we returned to civilization we became acutely aware of the social unrest nearby. There were riots going on in Los Angeles, and Rodney King's name had become immortalized. It was a strange experience to have been out of touch with the world's events for so long.

One of my Outward Bound instructors, Bill Liske, was an experienced guide in Nepal. We agreed we should do a trip together in the future. I arranged to meet Bill in Kathmandu on December 3, 1992. We were going to do a month-long trek through the Solu-Khumbu in Nepal. First I had to fly to Bangkok, where I would stay for a couple days until my flight to Kathmandu. When I got to the airport in Bangkok, a man from the tourist bureau took me aside and said the cab drivers were going to offer to take me to prostitutes. However, many were sick with AIDS, and I should avoid going. If I wanted to have sex...I stopped him there. I told him I just wanted to go to my hotel and relax. I had seen enough AIDS for a lifetime and had no desire to be exposed to any more.

I was shocked at the squalor of Kathmandu. It was a very sketchy, sad place. Dirty children played ball in the alleys. Poor people were everywhere. The only exception was the Grand Palace, the official residence of the Kings of Siam since the 1700s, which was opulent by contrast.

On our trek, we came across a few people who required the services of a doctor. I had brought some antibiotics with me and lanced a few abscesses. The sherpas and porters live in the mountains and come down for a few months during the trekking season to guide treks and carry supplies for the foreigners like me. Dawa Sherpa was our main guide. He spoke English very well, as he had spent a year as an instructor with Outward Bound in the United States. I told him about this new illness that was sweeping the world called AIDS, secondary to the HIV virus, and told him to tell the other sherpas to be careful whom they slept with when they went to Kathmandu.

We spent three days praying with the monks at the Tengbuche Monastery and celebrated the festival of Mani Rimdu. Mani Rimdu lasts for nineteen days. The last three days is a large festival where Nepalese and Tibetans gather from far and wide. It is a celebration of the establishment of Tibetan Buddhism. There are dancing, music, and hours of meditation. The temple is located more than 12,000 feet above sea level and is only accessed by the trekking trails. There are no roads. The Tibetans had to travel over very high mountain passes by foot to come—often in bare feet! They were quite distinctive: their skin was ruddy brown, their clothes were homemade, and their hair was wild.

After we bade the monks farewell and they gave us many prayer shawls for good luck, a wonderful custom, we climbed one of the sacred mountains of the Solu up to Dudh Kunda (Milky Lake) at 14,960 feet above sea level. We placed prayer flags we had brought with us in memory of a group of Outward Bound instructors who had been killed in an avalanche back in the LaSalle Mountains in southeast Utah, the site of my Outward Bound adventure.

Because we had left the main trekking trail, we were no longer sleeping in teahouses (residences that put up trekkers); we camped outside on the mountain. Bill and I shared a tent and the sherpas and porters shared the other two. One night after we had gone into our tents to go to sleep, Dawa came to my tent. He and the other sherpas and porters were so concerned, they could not go to sleep. They were worried they could catch AIDS by sleeping in the same tent together.

I reassured Dawa. I explained the transmission of the HIV virus in more detail: sleeping in the same tent with others was different than "sleeping" with a prostitute in Kathmandu.

15

SHARK ATTACK

I WAS AT the County on August 18, 1991, as a medical student doing my surgical rotation in trauma. For two weeks of the rotation, the medical students were part of the trauma team, basically responding to anything related to trauma that came through the ER. It was my turn to assist in the OR, on a patient with a stab wound to the chest. It was 10:30 p.m. when we entered the operating room. The patient was already intubated and the nurses had prepped and draped the patient's chest. I had never been part of a big trauma case before, and I was apprehensive.

I asked one of the nurses who the attending was, and she told me it was "Napoleon…the little dictator."

I knew she meant Dr. Tom Scalia, head of the surgical department. He looked about forty, just a little gray on the sides of a full head of hair, cropped short. He was short and thin, and he wore horn-rimmed glasses. Most of the nurses at the County were from the Caribbean and were quite large, on average about 250 pounds. The contrast was striking.

I had slept through a few of Dr. Scalia's lectures already. Not that he was boring, but after doing a thirty-hour shift, sitting in an uncomfortable wooden chair in a lecture hall across the street at Downstate with the lights dimmed, made it hard to stay awake. I hoped he hadn't noticed, and I hoped I hadn't snored.

We all knew how mean surgeons could be and were terrified by the phrases "shark rounds" and "morbidity and mortality conferences." These were like intellectual mixed martial arts matches with no holds barred. "Shark rounds" were held in the morning with the attending surgeon. The entire team would be assembled—from medical students, to interns, residents, and even the chief resident. We would discuss the current cases. The medical student du jour would present their case and be asked questions. We all bought books intended to help medical students and interns prepare for that moment, but being the focus of this circle of highly intelligent, aggressive doctors was intimidating.

Generally, the medical students would be able to handle a few questions, but when they got something wrong, the blood was in the water and at that point, the torture usually began. Unfortunately, doctors have been using this form of intellectual torture for years as standard boot camp-style training. It was done to them, so they are apt to do it to you. It doesn't matter if you were up all night holding a retractor in the OR on a 450-pound patient trying to keep their belly open enough for the resident to run the entire length of the bowel looking for a perforation.

I learned that if you answered about four questions correctly and confidently, the interrogator would move on to the next level, the interns, and ask them more challenging questions. This would go on all the way up to the PGY 4s (fourth-year postgraduates; you're designated by what level you were in the program, roughly correlating to how many years one has been out of medical school. If you don't do well, you may not advance to the next PGY. Or if you take time off to do research you would re-enter at the level you were when you left).

One of the first things we learn as students, and also probably the most common operation in the United States, is inguinal hernia surgery. We learn that there are three layers that the surgeon cuts through to access the hernia. Indirect hernias are more common (roughly two-thirds of all hernia surgeries) than direct hernias. I had read this many times and knew it could be asked of me and felt I was as ready as I could be for a swim with the sharks later this week.

On August 18th, I was told that I would be assisting in the operating room. Before you even get into the operating room, however, you must first run the scrub nurse's gauntlet. For the uninitiated (i.e., the med students), entering the OR is an adventure. First, you have to get into scrubs (if you aren't already in them), and don a mask and bonnet or cap. Then you need to open a scrub packet that contains a plastic pick in order to clean underneath your nails. The packet contains a plastic bristle brush on one side, and on the other, a sponge presoaked with a special cleaning solution. You need to wash up to above your elbows and really scrub your nails and fingers for several minutes.

Arms dripping wet, you enter the OR backward to avoid touching anything with your hands. A nurse who was already gowned and scrubbed in would then present a surgical gown. You insert your arms and get your hands through the white cuffs, and then you hold one end of a blue paper belt and turn around while the nurse holds the other end in order to close the back of the gown, allowing you to tie the belt. The nurse assists you with getting your gloves on. At any time, if you touched anything, the nurse would scowl at you and make you repeat the entire procedure all over again. It seemed like they took great pleasure in torturing the medical students and would make them re-scrub if they did even the slightest thing wrong.

I made it through the gauntlet of the scrub ritual eventually and stood next to a nurse on the patient's right side. Dr. Scalia entered the room a few minutes later with the chief resident. They were discussing other cases as they went through scrub, and then arrived at the operating table and began the surgery.

After cutting through the patient's skin, Dr. Scalia felt something and said, "What's this?" He continued to palpate and opened up a pocket where he showed me some tubing going vertically down the patient's right chest. I had no idea what it was.

He said rhetorically, "Didn't anyone check his chest X-ray?"

Of course we did—I mean *I* did, as did a few of the other residents. The guy had been shot in the chest! I went through the X-ray in my mind and could see the shrapnel. At the time, I had wondered what caliber the bullet was. There was a lot of white in the right chest, signifying blood. There was a punctured lung, which we thought measured about 33 percent at the apex. The heart seemed fine. There was a shattered right anterior rib. Nothing else stood out in my mind.

"You guys didn't look very closely at the X-ray. This is probably a V-P shunt," Dr. Scalia said. A ventriculoperitoneal catheter is tubing that connects from the patient's brain (lateral ventricle) through tubing that goes down the neck and chest and terminates in the belly. It is usually placed in patients who have obstruction of the brain's plumbing system (hydrocephalus). We had almost cut right through the tubing, which would have been a costly mistake for the patient.

After a few moments of silence, Dr. Scalia asked me a question. "Do you know the layers of the groin for inguinal hernia surgery?"

Holy shit! The inquisition is about to start! My brain started to race. I could barely think.

I answered firmly, "Yes." I didn't elaborate.

He continued with the surgery and did not address me again. He chatted with the chief resident as they proceeded to perform a right upper lobectomy. About an hour in, Dr. Scalia prodded the nurse standing next to me because she had fallen asleep. He seemed totally energized, while the rest of us were barely keeping awake. I stood there "assisting" for the next hour, trying to keep my eyes open.

The lung surgery was finished, and Dr. Scalia told the chief that he was going to take off. He had to give a lecture to the medical students (I was one of them) in a few hours and wanted to get some rest. The chief allowed me to help close the chest. The patient would go off to recovery. We tore off our gowns and masks and left the OR. It was 2:45 a.m. As we left the OR, my beeper went off and I was needed back down in the ER. I phoned down there, and my resident told me they needed me to run some blood samples to the lab immediately for type and cross (for a blood transfusion).

It sounded like I would be going back to the OR soon. Things were going crazy down there, and they needed all of us to help.

16

HISTORY REPEATS ITSELF

Kings County Hospital is located on Clarkson Avenue in Brooklyn. The neighborhood was largely populated by black people, most of whom had immigrated to the United States from Haiti. Many were poor. The other major population, which lived mostly on Eastern Parkway, was Hasidic Jews, most of whom were pretty successful. The Hasidic Jews are extremely religious and wear traditional black garb. They are easy to spot. The contrast between the two cultures couldn't have been more striking.

On my drive to work, I would pass a karate studio in the neighborhood, and there was a combination of Hasidic Jews with full beards, wearing karate gis over their traditional black suits, and young black men training together. Crazy!

At approximately 8:00 p.m. on August 19, 1991, a three-car motorcade for Rabbi Menachem Mendel Schneerson, leader of the Chabad Lubavitch Hasidic sect, was heading through the neighborhoods near the County. The procession was led by two officers in an unmarked police car with its rooftop light flashing.

One of the vehicles fell behind. Not wishing to lose the other motorcade vehicles, the laggard driver ran a red light. Unfortunately, the vehicle struck an oncoming car and went out of control up onto the sidewalk. The vehicle hit a building and pinned two black children against the iron grate covering the window. One of the two children was killed instantly, seven-year-old Gavin Cato. His seven-year-old cousin Angela Cato was severely injured.

The driver of the limo got out of the car and tried to help; however, a crowd of mostly black people formed at the accident scene. Some of the crowd started to beat the driver.

There is a special volunteer ambulance service for the Hasidic and Orthodox Jews called Hatzolah. The ambulance personnel are cognizant of the particulars of the Hasidic culture and try to provide emergency transport for Orthodox and Hasidic Jews. They are familiar with Jewish laws of modesty for females, rules for the Sabbath, and so forth. They are also noted for their rapid response times.

The Hatzolah ambulance arrived on the scene first. The medics attended to the injured children until the city ambulance arrived. The city paramedics told the Hatzolah medics to attend to the limo driver, and they would take care of the children. When the crowd, which had grown to about 250 people, saw the Hatzolah medics seemingly abandon the more seriously injured children, several began to chant anti-Semitic jeers.

Riots broke out shortly thereafter. Looting started that evening, directed against the Hasidic Jewish homes in the neighborhood. As with the current racial unrest in Ferguson, Missouri, the Reverend Al Sharpton was there to lead protest marches about the unjust treatment of blacks. One striking difference between then and now is the Reverend was much heavier in those days. Some of the leaders of the black community made anti-Semitic remarks and rallied the blacks against the Jews.

As the tensions built and the riots began, I was still inside the County, oblivious to the chaos outside.

The next day, four blocks from the event that led to Gavin Cato's death, a group of about twenty young black men surrounded a car stopped at a red light. The driver, Yankel Rosenbaum, a Hasidic Jew visiting from Australia to do research for his doctoral degree, was dragged from his car. He was beaten and stabbed by members of the angry mob. The police arrived and pursued the assailants. They apprehended a sixteen-year-old black youth named Lemrick Nelson Jr. who reportedly had a bloody knife in his pocket. Before Yankel was taken to the hospital, he identified Nelson as one of his assailants. (Years later, Nelson would admit he stabbed Yankel.)

Yankel was brought to Kings County Hospital ER, the only Level 1 Trauma Center in Brooklyn. However, the County had been neglected over the years, and the trauma room was not what most people think of as a modern hospital. It was a large room with areas for stretchers. There were no monitors hanging from the walls. There were none of the modern electronics that are associated with a first-world hospital. It was just a larger room with an ambulance entrance.

Although the EMTs had told the receiving residents in the ER he had been stabbed on both sides of his back, Yankel was quickly evaluated and felt to be stable by the residents on the trauma team. No chest X-ray was obtained during that first critical hour that Yankel was in the ER, the so-called "golden hour," when patients are deemed to be most salvageable after trauma.

Mayor David Dinkins, the city's first black mayor, came to the County ED with an entourage to help quell the riots. They even stopped to see Yankel during their visit, shortly before he went into shock and died. It was reported that he died from internal bleeding from one of his chest wounds. Presumably he had a hemothorax—bleeding into the chest cavity (which can hold several liters of blood). A chest X-ray for patients with stab wounds to the chest was standard, even back in the old days. A patient is likely to have a pneumothorax (punctured lung) when anything sharp enters the chest. A pneumothorax can be life-threatening in and of itself, even if there is no bleeding. A chest X-ray is a fast and accurate way of figuring out if there is a punctured lung and how much bleeding there is in the chest.

The combination of bleeding around the lung and a punctured lung (hemopneumothorax) often necessitates placing a tube into the chest to drain the blood and air out to allow the lung to expand and take in oxygen. If the bloody drainage is significant, patients are often taken immediately to the OR to find the source of bleeding and to stop it so the patient won't bleed to death. Other options are to go to the angiography suite and have the interventional radiologist try to plug up the bleeding from the inside. At any rate, significant bleeding into the chest is a very bad thing and needs to be recognized and treated immediately. Being surprised by this and delaying the patient's care by not recognizing a hemopneumothorax can easily be a fatal mistake, and in Yankel's case, it was.

For several days, riots ensued. The following evening, when I was heading back to work after sleeping for a few hours at home, I found the tires on my car were slashed. I rode my bike to work.

Hundreds of riot police lined Eastern Parkway for days. They held large plastic shields and wore helmets. They had batons at the ready. It felt like a war zone. Rioters battled with police, and at one point, the police had to retreat. The riots and looting lasted for three days, during which many people were injured. We were inundated with patients, as most victims were brought to the County. I saw more serious injuries in the two weeks on that rotation than many ER docs see in a decade.

About two weeks after the riots subsided, a man from Italy was driving in the neighborhood near the hospital. A group of black men surrounded his car, and one of them shot and killed him. He had a white beard and was dressed in dark business attire, similar to what the Hasidic Jews would wear.

The driver of the car that killed Gavin Cato was not indicted.

And although Lemrick Nelson apparently confessed to the crime to police at the time of his arrest, and also confessed at his third trial in 2003 and apologized to Yankel's family, he was never convicted of Yankel's murder. He was also unsuccessfully tried for a hate crime. Ultimately, Lemrick was convicted of violating Yankel's civil rights and served ten years in prison. Since that time, Lemrick has had several additional run-ins with the law. In 2010, he was himself the victim of a stabbing, by an icepick to his skull.°≠≠≠

17

JURY DUTY

A s OF JANUARY 1996, the City of New York tightened the exemptions for serving jury duty, and doctors were no longer
exempt.[7] I was asked to serve and had no choice but to accept. I
was co–chief resident and on backup call for everything. If anyone was out or needed help at any time of day, Tommy and I were
the backups for all thirty other residents. It seemed unfathomable
that I would have to turn my beeper off. I had never heard of resident physicians being called for jury duty, and we had no official
administrative classification to account for it. Would it count as
vacation time?

I had never missed a day of work except for going to my grandfather's funeral four years earlier when I was an intern.[8] I talked to
my director, and he said I should tell them, as chief resident, I am
essential to Kings County Hospital, that my beeper was always on,
and that I couldn't miss any time from work.

I showed up at the Brooklyn Courthouse and sat down in a
large auditorium with hundreds of other potential jurors. Guards

---

7 Debra M. Katz, "Exemptions for Jury Duty Tightened," *New York Times*,
January 7, 1996.
8 See Chapter 4: Pacemaker

were placed at the door. At 9:00 a.m., they closed the doors behind the guards.

A speaker announced, "Anyone who does not speak English may leave now."

About a third of the potential jurors got up immediately and began to leave. I chuckled to myself. *Uh, if they didn't speak English, how did they understand what he said so quickly?* It seemed like a trick.

The rest of us sat in the wooden chairs awaiting our fate. Our names were called, and we were shuttled off to different rooms by armed guards. In the first jury selection, for an armed-robbery trial, the lawyer for the defense, a well-put-together woman about my age, began asking me questions.

"Mr. Stoane, you are a doctor in training. Correct?"

She said it laced with venom, and it sounded like I used training wheels. "Yes. However, I prefer to be addressed as either Dr. Stoane or Jason."

"Mr. Stoane—" she said as she started to ask another question, but I interrupted her.

"Just call me Dr. Stoane."

"Mr. Jason, have you ever been robbed?"

Is she for real? I thought. *Is she trying to get under my skin?*

The lawyer for the prosecution could see that this was becoming a bad situation and said, "Judge, she doesn't need to continue with the witness. We don't want him."

I was dismissed from that jury.

I went back to the main room and waited to hear my name called again.

The next jury I almost sat on was for a case about a person who had fallen in a hospital elevator and broke his leg. The lawyer for the defense tried to get me dismissed right away because I worked for a hospital. (It seemed clear to me that the system was not quite ready to handle doctors as jurors.) The judge told the defense attorney that even he could get called for jury duty, so I would have to stay. He began to argue with the lawyer and then the judge addressed me personally.

"Dr. Stoane, we need you to put aside your training as a physician and be a layperson. You are to listen to the experts and accept what they say as the expert. You are not allowed to answer medical questions for your peers. Are you able to do that?"

I was taken aback. All my training, over the past ten years, had been to think critically about medical situations. Doctors looked to me for help and advice on their patients all the time. Radiologists interpret X-rays, CT scans, MRIs, ultrasounds, PET scans, and mammograms, and discuss their impressions with the doctors who order the studies. We are often asked for advice to help figure out what is going on with those doctors' patients. Our most important roles are as diagnosticians and consultants. And the judge was asking me to shut it all off for this case.

I answered, "Judge, would it be possible for you to stop being a judge for a trial?"

He shot back, "Can you or can't you be a doctor?"

"Judge, with all due respect, this is who I am. I don't think I can just turn off all the years of study and training."

The lawyer for the defense chimed in, saying, "Judge, we do not want to seat Dr. Stoane."

I was dismissed again.

The last jury selection I was dismissed from was a rape trial that was definitely going to be sequestered. I really did not want to be sequestered and was scrambling to figure out a way to get out of it. Many of the other jurors were either retired or unemployed. I needed to get back to work!

"Mr. Stoane, have you ever treated a rape victim?" The lawyer for the defense asked.

"Yes," I responded, deadpan.

Here we go again. Perhaps they don't understand that a resident physician is a real doctor with a real MD. I graduated from medical school four years ago! I screamed in my brain.

"Did you have any negative feelings for the person who raped your patient?" He asked.

"Of course!" I said.

"Judge, we won't need Mr. Stoane."

I was dismissed again. Once I was back in the auditorium, a guard informed us it was getting late and that we were dismissed for the day. Our civil-service duty was done.

Glad that was over. I was exhausted but relieved. I didn't realize how anxious I had been all day. I felt like I was on trial, the way I was treated. *So much for doing my civic duty.* I felt like I had escaped the frying pan. Now, back to the fire.

18

GETTING STUCK

W HEN I STARTED at Downstate as a medical student, I had heard that a young doctor had gotten the new plague, AIDS, from a needle stick at the County. Dr. Veronica Prego was an intern who claimed she got AIDS when she was accidentally infected by a needle left at her patient's bedside by another doctor after a blood draw.[9] She sued the city of New York for over $100 million for negligence. The case ultimately settled for $1.35 million. She went on to complete a gastroenterology fellowship and appears to be still practicing today—a miracle, considering most people I knew and cared for who contracted HIV in the 1980s died with AIDS.

We were all terrified of catching the HIV virus. We had no blood-draw teams or IV teams. The interns and residents put themselves in harm's way all the time. After Dr. Prego's suit, the hospital added red disposal boxes in all patient rooms to place all the needles (aka "sharps").

We would double-glove, but when we were suturing, it was not uncommon to get stuck by a dirty needle. I was fortunate I was taught how to handle sharps well, and the only time I got stuck

9 Arnold H. Lubasch, "Settlement Ends Prego Trial on Brink of Summations," *New York Times*, March 9, 1990.

by a dirty needle in the nine years I was at the County was when I was doing a lumbar puncture and myelogram (injecting dye into the sack around the spinal cord under X-ray guidance) on an eighty-two-year-old woman. She needed a myelogram to exclude cord compression because an MRI was unavailable at night at the County. I was performing the exam with the assistance of a tech, but it was difficult to keep the patient positioned correctly, and I became distracted and accidentally stuck myself. I finished the exam.

I reviewed her chart and felt she was at low risk for infectious diseases, and I never reported the incident, as, I am certain, happened most of the time at the County.

19

Don't Tell Her
She Has AIDS!

M Y PATIENT WAS a young Caribbean woman who looked healthy. She was twenty-four years old and mildly obese. She came to the County ER with a cough that wouldn't go away. A chest X-ray was obtained, and it was interpreted by the radiology resident as "increased interstitial markings. Findings consistent with an interstitial pneumonitis, possible PCP." PCP, or pneumocystis pneumonia, is an opportunistic infection that affects only people with weakened immune systems. There are a few reasons to have an opportunistic infection, but the most common one in Brooklyn in the 1990s was AIDS.

We were told by our attending that we were not allowed to order HIV tests on our patients because there were new regulations from the State of New York that required post-test counseling for patients.[10] We needed to send the patient's blood off-site to get tested, and it could take a week or two to get the results back. By then, the patient might have been discharged, and the residents and interns would probably have rotated onto different services.

---

10 I was unable to find any reference to this policy.

There was no guarantee that the patient would get the mandatory counseling, and the attending felt he would be on the hook to take care of all the counseling himself.

So, the solution was to not test our patients until there were better systems in place to ensure that we could meet the requirements.

At the time, there were resources that patients with AIDS could access: counseling, free medications, drug trials. It was imperative to make the diagnosis as early as possible, not just treat the infections. There were AIDS-defining diagnoses, which would qualify patients for the additional resources even if they did not have a positive HIV blood test. PCP pneumonia and other opportunistic infections, like toxoplasmosis in the brain in an otherwise healthy individual (not one who was on chemotherapy for a cancer which would impair their immune system), were acceptable. In addition, invasive cervical cancer and Kaposi's sarcoma were qualifying.

Kaposi's sarcoma was seen less frequently in our patient population at the County and seemed more common in gay men, who were more prevalent at hospitals in Manhattan. Our patients were more likely to have PCP pneumonia, toxoplasmosis in the brain, and drug-resistant TB (tuberculosis).

Our patient was overweight, like many of the Caribbean women who live in Crown Heights, and had a full head of kinky hair. Becoming unnaturally thin and the straightening of a black person's hair are telltale signs of AIDS at the County. She was robust and didn't look sick at all. The only abnormality in her labs was that her partial thromboplastin time (PTT) was abnormally high. This is one of the measures of the ability of a person's blood to form clots. It turns out that many HIV-positive patients make a protein (lupus anticoagulant[11]) that inhibits clotting and increasing of the PTT. We would use this fact to bolster the argument that she probably had PCP pneumonia and underlying HIV.

---

11 Franklin A. Bontempo, MD, "The Lupus Anticoagulant—An Update," Institute for Transfusion Medicine, May 2001, http://www.itxm.org/tmu/tmu2001/tmu5-2001.htm.

The test that would be most helpful, in lieu of an HIV test, was a CD4/CD8 test, which would tell us whether her T-cells— immune cells—were compromised by the HIV infection. A very low CD4 count (less than 50) would indicate a severely immuno-compromised patient who would be susceptible to opportunistic infections (infections that her body could ordinarily wipe out or suppress without breaking a sweat).

To make the diagnosis of PCP pneumonia, the chest X-ray needed to be suspicious. PCP pneumonia looks different than regular bacterial pneumonia. Bacterial pneumonia tends to give a region of increased density or whiteness on the chest X-ray. PCP pneumonia gives thickening of the interstitial lines on the X-ray emanating from the center to the periphery. The lungs look dirty.

Oftentimes, the patients presented with a cough or low-grade fever. They looked normal— healthy. PCP pneumonia does not look any different from the "walking pneumonia" that healthy people get, which can be treated with erythromycin. PCP responds best to Bactrim, a drug that costs pennies and has been around for years. However, Bactrim can have severe side effects, particularly in black patients (with a genetic disorder called G6PD deficiency), so we had to be judicious in prescribing it.

Making the diagnosis of PCP pneumonia involved the patient undergoing a fairly invasive procedure called a bronchoscopy, where a scope is inserted down the airway by a pulmonologist and samples of cells are taken from deep in the lung. The patient is usually heavily sedated during the procedure, to tolerate the "snake" going down their trachea. The samples are examined in the pathology lab, and the diagnosis is made by identifying inclusion cysts within the lung cells, which are characteristic for this infection.

I had consulted the psychiatry service, because when I was discussing what I thought was going on with the patient, and saying I wanted her to get bronchoscoped, she told me in no uncertain terms that she would kill herself if I told her she had AIDS. I thought she was being hyperbolic, but I didn't feel I could ignore what she said, either. She didn't seem in the least bit depressed, but when I probed further, she said she would "jump right through that window, if you tell me I have AIDS." She pointed to the window behind me. (We were on the eighth floor of the County on A72.)

I was fully aware of the recent incident where a mentally ill patient had jumped off the sixth floor of G Building, and was killed by the fall, and I didn't want to take any chances.[12]

The attending psych floored me. "Do not tell her, under any circumstances, that she has AIDS." That was his professional advice.

I asked him, "What if the bronchoscopy results come back as positive for PCP pneumonia? It's an AIDS-defining diagnosis."

He repeated, "Do not tell her she has AIDS. You don't even have an HIV test, do you? Tell her she has PCP pneumonia and treat her for it." He finished the note in her chart, left the chart room, and headed for the elevator.

I followed him to the elevator and argued it would be important for her to get AIDS-related services, medications, and counseling. I told him I didn't feel comfortable withholding important information from the patient.

He retorted, "Do no harm, Doctor!"

"She needs to know," I responded. "This seems so paternal."

"You don't have an HIV test, so you therefore can't say for certain that she has HIV. Can you?" he said. "I am telling you that you should not tell her she has AIDS unless you have definitive proof. Since you cannot order an HIV test at this time, then you cannot, and should not, put her life in jeopardy by telling her she has AIDS. That is my final opinion on the subject!"

---

12 Josh Barbanel, "Patient at Kings County Dies in Plunge, Police Report," *New York Times*, October 8, 1991.

I stood there completely flummoxed, but did not have time to process the information.

She got bronchoscoped the next day and the results came back the following day that she had PCP pneumonia. I started her on Bactrim. Every day on rounds she would ask me what her diagnosis was and when she could go home. Each day, I tried to avoid her. She knew. She was just trying to force me to say it.

On Thursday, I called her mother and asked her to come in to the hospital so she could pick up her daughter and we could all talk. I told her mom that she had recovered nicely and was ready for discharge. I had decided that I would recommend to the two of them that, as an outpatient, she should, among other things, get an HIV test, which her doctor could order, just to be on the safe side.

On Friday morning's rounds, my patient decided to corner me. She was my height, but outweighed me by about seventy pounds. As I was finishing up with another patient, she had come up behind me and had basically pinned me against the wall, next to the bed.

She said, "I want to know, *now*! I want to know if I have AIDS!"

I was stuck. Both physically and mentally.

"Your mom will be here in a few hours and I will go over everything with you both at that time," I responded.

She persisted, "I want to know *now*!"

"Don't you think it will be better if we talk about all this when your mom is here with you?

"Tell me *now*! I need to know! I have a right to know!"

She had me. I thought she should know. I couldn't lie to her and I had tried to avoid telling her for several days. I submitted.

"Yes, I believe you have AIDS. You have an AIDS-defining diagnosis, PCP pneumonia. Only severely immunocompromised patients get this type of pneumonia. I am unable to get an HIV test now, so I recommend that you get one as soon as possible when you come in for your outpatient follow-up appointment."

Her eyes popped open, she raised her arms over her head, and she began screaming like a banshee as she headed out of the room and down the hallway. I ran after her to calm her down, but before I could reach her, she ran into the elevator and the door closed.

I ran back to the nursing station and told the nurse to call security. I also sheepishly put in an emergency call to psychiatry.

Security captured her before she left the building. They brought her back up to her room. She was exhausted, but still weeping. I told her I would call her mother and she thanked me.

The attending psych arrived a few moments later and berated me. "I told you not to tell her. Now, you've told her and I need to clean up the mess you created."

I apologized and thanked him for coming to help. He prescribed her some medications that calmed her down. I had a long conference with her and her mother before discharging her that afternoon.

20

NOT AGAIN!

I WALKED DOWN the hallway to A72. I had a thirty-two-year-old patient, Mr. Dubois, with HIV and TB. He had miliary TB, which spread to his brain. He had been treated for two months and was recovering. He was conscious, but his thought processes were slowed and it was difficult to assess him because he only spoke Haitian Creole.

His main medical problem at this point was a recurrent pleural effusion (fluid around the lung). It was probably due to irritation of the lining of the lung from the TB. I needed to check the amount of fluid every day. Instead of getting him a chest X-ray and exposing him to radiation daily, my dad told me about a method where I could monitor his effusion clinically. He told me to have the patient sit up in the same position every day when I examined him, put my stethoscope on his back, and percuss (tap) my finger on his back. The sound would change when I tapped over a normal lung versus when I tapped over fluid. I would then mark his back with a magic marker. Ingenious!

Like many of my patients from Haiti, the patient had no visitors. Today, however, there was a well-dressed older couple standing at the foot of his bed having a conversation with Mr. Dubois. I was ecstatic to finally meet his parents! I started to tell them how much better he was in comparison to when he was admitted. I told him the TB infection was under control and I thought he would be ready for discharge soon. I went on to tell them his HIV infection was under control for now.

They stopped me. "We are not his parents. We are his aunt and uncle. We did not know he had HIV. No one in the family knew that!"

Crap! I just did it again!

21

I'm Not Dead Yet

"I'LL TAKE THESE three patients, and you go and work up the hi-fiver with anemia in the prison ward."

"Hi-fiver" was slang for an HIV-positive patient (V is the Roman numeral for five). I was trying to get rid of my annoying medical student for a while so I could work on the more complicated patients who were admitted to me.

Actually, it wasn't that he was annoying; he was just really slow. If I had learned anything, it was to be efficient. If I ever expected to leave the building, I had to work and think fast. How hard could it be to take a history and do a physical on a prisoner with AIDS and anemia?

It seemed like a good idea at the time because the three "hits" I had were not easy. I took their history and did their physicals, got their blood drawn, tracked down their X-rays, and wrote my notes. I ran the blood down to the lab. My resident was on the other team, so he spent all his time helping his intern. It would make their job easier in the morning. I would have liked to have the help too, but such is life. I even started to write discharge notes on two of the three patients. The third patient was still an unknown to me, so that one could wait until we got the labs back and went over him with my resident in the morning. Time to track down that pesky third-year medical student.

When prisoners from Rikers Island need inpatient care, they are transported to B31, the twenty-six-bed prison ward at Kings County Hospital. To enter the ward, you need to press a big red button on the wall next to the right side of the door to be granted entrance. There's a camera next to the door, and you need to show the guard your ID by holding it up to the camera. The big steel door is opened remotely, allowing you to step inside. The door closes behind you, and now you are between the door and two sets of prison bar doors, which create a cage of sorts. The same guard will then press a button that opens the first set of bar doors. A buzz sounds and the door opens, and then you step inside the cage. Another guard sits behind bulletproof glass. After another ID check, the guard decides whether you are acceptable, and will press a button and buzz you through the second set of bar doors to finally enter the prison ward. It's the same procedure in reverse when you want to leave.

I always found all the scrutiny to be over the top. How many short, balding white guys in a white doctors coat with a stethoscope sticking out of his pocket have ever tried to break into a hospital prison ward?

I made it through the Maxwell Smart–like security check and found my MS 3 standing at the foot of the patient's bed. It was a bizarre scene: the med student was trying to take a history, but the patient looked barely conscious. He was speaking gibberish, but the student didn't seem to notice.

I interrupted, exclaiming, "How come you didn't page me? This guy is really sick! What the hell...I thought he just had anemia!"

I grabbed the chart from my student and looked at the patient's initial set of labs, which had been obtained while the patient had been in the ER. I realized the first mistake. The results had been transposed.[13] His HCT was abnormally high because he was extremely dehydrated and his blood cells were very thick. He was so dehydrated, his blood sugar level was 400 (normal is less than 100); he was entering a diabetic coma. Also, his corrected sodium level (the amount of sodium in the bloodstream needs to be recalculated when the blood sugar is high) was incredibly low, a really bad sign. They completely missed the boat in the ED. This guy was really sick and needed to be in the ICU, not stuck in the prison ward. Fortunately, someone in the ED had found a vein in which to place an IV and had started IV fluids. The patient was also an intravenous drug abuser and had no good veins left for us from which to draw blood.

The best way to treat a diabetic coma is to give lots of fluids and insulin. High sugar levels cause patients to urinate away most of their body water. Correcting the high sugar and restoring the normal concentration of fluids is paramount. However, we needed to correct his low sodium as well, very slowly. One of the dreaded complications of correcting the sodium too quickly is central pontine myelinolysis. The neurons in the central pons, a portion of the brainstem, are very sensitive to rapid changes in sodium levels, and if the levels change rapidly, the cells can die. If a patient develops this syndrome, they could lose all kinds of neurological function, and end up in a "locked-in" condition. When a patient is "locked-in," it means they are totally paralyzed, except for the muscles around their eyes. I had seen a patient get locked in after he had a clot travel from his heart to his brain's basilar artery. The only thing he could do was blink.

The rate at which blood sodium levels can return to normal is quite variable. The only way to monitor this rate is to constantly

---

13 His HCT (hematocrit, the amount of fluid volume in the bloodstream) wasn't 14—that was his Hgb result (hemoglobin, the molecules that actually transport oxygen). The ratio is 3:1 (Hgb:HCT), so his HCT was actually 52 instead of 14. An HCT level of 52 is abnormally high (between 40 and 44 is considered normal), and certainly not anemic.

test the patient's blood (at least once an hour) and regularly adjust the amount of fluids and the contents of the fluids, as necessary. Today, we have handheld machines made initially for the military that can take a drop of blood and test it at the patient's bedside in about a minute. The early 1990s was prehistoric in comparison. Besides having to navigate the labyrinth to get in and out of the prison ward each time, we needed to hand deliver the samples to the lab, which wasn't even in the same building as the patients.

The pathology building was connected to B Building by a bridge and the laboratory was on the ground floor, three floors down. There was no vacuum-tube system that could send the samples long distances quickly. Each slip needed to be filled out by hand, and the patient's ID info was stamped onto the lab slip. At that time, there were no IV teams, phlebotomy teams, or expert blood drawers to magically descend on a patient as soon as the doctor wrote the order. The residents, interns, and med students performed all these tasks.

Trying to correct this patient's sodium in the prison ward seemed an impossible task. I called the resident I was working with and could almost hear him smirk on the other end of the phone. He said he would talk to the chief resident about trying to move him to the ICU. But he thought it would be a waste of time: the patient had AIDS, diabetic ketoacidosis, and a severe electrolyte imbalance that was life-threatening. He was not salvageable and they needed the ICU beds for patients who were.

Since he was so dehydrated and an intravenous drug abuser, he had no good veins from which we could draw blood. Since we were not in the unit, we weren't allowed to place a central venous catheter. So, each time we needed blood, we had to puncture his femoral veins. I guessed this was as good a time as any to teach my medical student something useful. I showed him how to feel for the femoral artery and go toward the inner thigh for it. I taught him the mnemonic for the femoral triangle (groin)—NAVL (nerve, artery, vein, lymph)—from lateral to medial. I also had the opportunity to teach him to be very vigilant about the handling of needles. Since most of our patients had HIV, we needed to be extra cautious about this process. We were told to never recap a needle with our fingers. We were responsible for disposing of our sharps in the red containers when we were finished.

Puncturing the groin is painful, but we had no choice, and the patient was not cognizant of what we were doing anymore. We had to get the lab slips ready by impressing his card with his information, checking off the labs we wanted run, and grabbing the appropriate tubes (red tops) and the venipuncture material (alcohol wipes, gauze, tape, needles, and specimen bags). The first time, I showed him how I did it. (We had a saying, "See one, do one, teach one.") Then one of us needed to run the blood down to the lab by going through the series of the prison-ward doors.

Fortunately, we had IV access via one of his external jugular veins in his neck. We hung the bags of IV fluids on a pole and titrated the amounts of insulin, sodium, and potassium based on his labs, which we sent off every hour or so starting at 9:00 p.m. I asked the resident if we had gotten approval for an ICU transfer, and he told me there were no beds. I asked him to check again in the morning, if the patient was still alive.

We took turns running the specimens to the lab all night.

In the morning, we presented the patient to our resident and attending. We showed them the chart of his sodium and glucose. His sodium was still abnormal, but we were a lot closer to normal. We had not gone too fast with the correction, and it was unlikely we had fried his brain. His glucose still seemed difficult to control. Our attending praised our efforts and told us he would push for the patient to be transferred to the ICU. We continued our hourly blood draws, and he was transferred to the unit by 2:00 p.m.

I was totally spent. I sent my medical student home. I wrote my progress notes and finished up as much as I could on my other eleven patients. Finally, I got home by 7:00 p.m. and collapsed.

Two weeks later, I got a call from the resident.

"Guess who's bouncing back to you?" he said, with a little too much glee in his voice. "Mr. DKA [diabetic ketoacidosis], who you sent to the unit. Oh, and you missed his diagnosis. The chief wants to talk to you about that, by the way."

"What did I miss?" I said, becoming angry and defensive.

"The reason why he went into DKA. You never figured out why he went into DKA," the resident said.

My mind was scrambling. *What did I miss?* I was so busy trying to fix his sodium and his sugar levels. I just thought he was an uncontrolled diabetic.

"He was never a diabetic before this incident," the resident said, toying with me. "You missed that he had a fever."

"A fever?" I tried to recall his chart, but remembered only his sodium and sugar problems.

"Yes. He had a low-grade fever, and in the ICU they performed a lumbar puncture and found he had meningitis. Candida meningitis!"

I had been so focused on his other problems, I missed a critical abnormality. *Fever!* Fever in a patient with AIDS always got a full-court press, because AIDS patients are susceptible to life-threatening, opportunistic infections, and they need to be treated quickly with the correct drugs. Candida is a fungus. Fungus in the spinal fluid that bathes the brain and spinal cord is a really bad thing. Only patients who have no immune systems get fungus in the cerebrospinal fluid and virtually all AIDS patients with candida meningitis die.

So, how did my patient survive with all of these problems? They gave him amphotericin, a very powerful antifungal medication, which we called "ampho-terrible." It can only be given intravenously and causes a depletion of magnesium. You need one IV line for the ampho and another one for the magnesium and IV fluids.

My patient came to in the ICU and was delusional. He had threatened to kill all the staff, so they had placed him in four-point limb restraints and had two prison guards at his bedside at all times. When a patient you send to the ICU gets well enough to go back out to the floor for care, the patient goes back to the doctor who originally treated him (same goes if you discharge a patient from the hospital and they get readmitted within the same calendar month). This is called a "bounce back."

My patient bounced back to my service when he was no longer critical. However, he still needed to have two IVs at all times and was in four-point restraints with the guards at his bedside at all times. The chief decided the patient was too difficult to take care of in the prison ward, so he was placed in a private room on A71. He had developed a decubitus ulcer (bedsore) on his back while in the ICU that was quite painful and difficult to take care of because he was in four-point restraints.

When I entered his room to evaluate him, the odor from the decubitus ulcer was overwhelming. The guards wore masks. He looked terrible. His eyes were half open. His mouth was open, and he had only a few teeth left. He had prison tattoos all over his body. His IVs were tenuously attached to his neck, and seemed ready to fail at any moment. He was contorting his body to get off his decubitus ulcer. I asked the guards if they would take his restraints off, and they said he was too dangerous.

"He's a bad man," one of them said.

I considered the situation and, exasperated, I said, "I can't take care of him. There's no way! He needs to be in the unit! He should be dead!"

At that point, the patient opened his eyes and said, "What's the problem, Doc? I'm not dead yet, and I'm not that sick! I want to go back to jail and get out of this place. "

"Those guys in the ICU were assholes, and if I see any one of them, I'll slit their throats! You were the one who took care of me when I came in, right? You did a good job, and I need you to get me out of here."

22

OFFICER DOWN!

THE FIRST PATIENT arrived in the ED within minutes of the incident. We had gotten a call from the dispatcher that there had been a shooting in the outpatient-clinic building only moments before.

The outpatient-clinic building was next to A Building and about a quarter-mile from the ED. It should only take a few minutes to transfer victims from there to the ED by ambulance. It might even be faster to just put them on a stretcher and run them over.

The first patient was a middle-aged corrections officer. He had been shot twice in the abdomen or lower chest. He was experiencing symptoms of shock, but he was conscious when he came in. We would get X-rays to try to figure out where the bullets were, and the patient would then go straight to the OR for exploration and repair of whatever was bleeding. This was pretty standard fare for the County. We lived in violent times, in large part due to drugs like crack cocaine.

We called it the "knife and gun" club. Guys would come in off the street and say, "I was just hanging out with the crowd, and I felt this stinging sensation in my leg. I looked down and I was bleeding." He was shot! Wrong place, wrong time.

We waited for the second patient. It seemed like a really long time between when the officer came in and when the prisoner got to us. When he finally did, he was dying, almost dead.

The prisoner had committed armed robbery just two days before. He and his accomplice unfortunately picked on the wrong guy, an off-duty corrections officer. The officer had just withdrawn money from an ATM when the two perpetrators blocked his way with their motorcycle and demanded the money. The officer gave them the money and then pulled out his weapon, and a gunfight ensued.

The prisoner's partner in crime was shot and killed during the robbery. Our patient was shot in the upper arm, but not seriously injured. He was well enough to be booked into jail. He was brought over to the orthopedics outpatient clinic for X-rays and to evaluate the bandage. Because he was deemed highly dangerous, his hands were shackled to his waist, and his feet were also shackled. The officers refused to unshackle him for the exam, which would have been a violation of protocol. At that point, the patient refused to be evaluated further.

The next day, the prisoner complained again and was brought by a different set of officers to the outpatient-clinic building to be examined. This time, they did unshackle him. He surprised them and overpowered one of the officers, grabbed her gun, and shot her partner twice. Her partner toppled to the ground. The prisoner tried to run down the hallway to escape, but couldn't move very fast because of the shackles binding his feet. The uninjured officer grabbed her downed partner's gun and ran down the hallway. The prisoner turned and fired at her twice, missing both times. She fired her borrowed weapon at him and hit him in the chest. He fell to the ground, seriously wounded.[14]

---

14 Ronald Sullivan, "Union Faults Correction Dept. in Shootout at Kings Hospital," *New York Times*, June 23, 1994.

I'm not certain the delay in transportation was purposefully done, but it might have reduced his chance of survival. The contrast between the transport times of the two victims seemed to speak volumes. We have a saying that it is usually the good guys who die and the bad ones who seem to always make it. Not this time.

23

JIUJITSU IN THE ER

A MARTIAL ARTS instructor began teaching classes at my gym. I became interested, and after about a year, I started training. I met my best friend there, Mitch. Neither of us was very talented, but we both worked hard to become proficient. We took additional instruction in boxing and jiujitsu over the years to improve our skills. To qualify for the black belt in our dojo (martial arts school), we needed to teach a karate class for one year. Our sensei (instructor) started a new dojo at a gym in Brooklyn Heights, and Mitch and I taught karate there together. After our workouts, we would head to Aunt Suzie's Restaurant for dinner in the Slope (Park Slope). There were two portion sizes at Aunt Suzie's: small size; and regular size, which the menu said would feed two yuppies.

I was standing in front of "the book" in the ED. The book was a well-worn red binder listing the patients who were to be admitted to the medical service each day. I was looking for my next patient to admit. Next to me were two New York City police officers. Most police officers I met were large individuals, and when they were decked out in their gear, they were pretty imposing. These officers were sitting at the bed of their prisoner, who was to be examined and probably admitted.

Out of the corner of my eye, I watched Claude, one of the ER attendings and a large man (six feet, 250 pounds), approaching a patient's bed about ten feet away. The patient, an older white man and probably homeless, was sleeping with the head of the bed propped up. Claude approached the bed with a syringe in his right hand. He was holding onto the patient's IV tubing in his left hand. An alarm sounded from the IV machine attached to the tubing, indicating that the IV was clogged. Before Claude could insert the needle into the IV tubing port to flush the line, the patient woke up and was startled by Claude's presence. The patient must have thought Claude was going to stab him, or he was so disoriented he didn't know what was going on. He grabbed Claude's throat with both hands and began to wring his neck. Claude didn't seem too bothered by the neck wringing, but seemed to be trying to avoid accidentally stabbing the patient with the needle, which was shaking wildly in his hand.

At first I was only vaguely aware of what was happening, but when it was clear that Claude was in trouble, I looked directly at the two large police officers decked out with bulletproof vests, 9 mm Glock handguns, and handcuffs, among other things. They looked at me and pointed to their charge and indicated with a shrug that Claude was my problem, not theirs. The officers did not want to leave their post or be distracted from their primary responsibility, guarding their inmate.[15]

Since no one seemed to be jumping in to help Claude, I decided to act. Claude was on the patient's right side, still waving the needle, so I chose the left side of the bed. I wrested the patient's left hand off Claude's neck and was able to bend his wrist in on itself and secure his elbow as I simultaneously wrapped my right arm around the back of his neck. I was basically lying on the gurney, trapping his left wrist in a bad spot. If he tried to move, I subdued

---

15 Craig Wolff, "Inmate Escapes from Hospital, Rapes Woman," *New York Times*, November 3, 1989.

him by increasing the pressure on his wrist. I could have easily put him in a chokehold with my right elbow, if necessary. However, even through his agitation and stupor, the pain in his wrist clearly caught his attention and he let go of Claude's throat. He tried to hit me with his right arm and squirm away from me, but I had pretty good control of him, and the more he moved, the more pressure I applied with my wristlock.

The whole series of events took about a minute. It seemed like an eternity with my head against the patient's neck, smelling his breath; a combination of alcohol and seemingly not having brushed his teeth for a month almost made me vomit. Four burly security officers eventually relieved me. It was amusing, because each one took an extremity, but he could still move them all, and the officers were unable to control him as he fought them for all he was worth for the next ten minutes, until he exhausted himself.

I dusted myself off and walked back over to the book, chuckling to myself. I had lost a button on my white coat. The two cops gave me the thumbs-up to sheepishly acknowledge my efforts and got back to focusing on the patient.

Another time for me to use my karate arose when I came in one morning at 7:45 a.m. and saw Pauli. Normally, he would have been on his way home from a long night shift. I saw Pauli at the angiography console reviewing images he had just obtained. He had just inserted a catheter into his patient's femoral artery and advanced a catheter into the aorta in the chest. He had just walked out of the angio room, with blood caked on his gloves. He concentrated so hard, he forgot about the blood and he held his gloved hand against his chin.

"Pauli, your glove?" I said.

"Oh," he said, distracted.

Pauli was reviewing an angio he was in the process of performing. It was an aortogram. The patient was a forty-eight-year-old Haitian man who had presented to the ED with chest and back pain. The CT scan was abnormal and showed a mass adjacent to the aorta, which Pauli thought was a clot from an aortic dissection. The surgery team wanted confirmation before they decided what course of action to take. The patient's vital signs were stable and they requested an angiogram.

"What's up?" I asked.

"I can't figure out where this contrast is going," he said. He touched the screen with his bloody glove.

"Pauli, your freaking glove!" I cried.

"Holy shit!" Pauli yelled.

At that very moment, both Pauli and I looked up, and through the glass window we saw the patient sit up and start to pull on the catheter and get off the angio table. Pauli ran to the side where the catheter was and tried to get the patient's hand away from it. The catheter was in his femoral artery and if he pulled it out, it would be disastrous.

I went to the head of the bed to try to hold him down. I grabbed his left hand and arm, and I used a wrist and elbow lock in order to distract him from grabbing the catheter. Although he was a large, strong man who was clearly delirious, I had a secure-enough lock that he gave up trying to rip the catheter out of his groin; it had already come almost all the way out.

The patient started to lose consciousness a moment later. Both Pauli and I realized now that what we had observed on the screen was an active aortic rupture. The contrast he injected was going from the aorta into the patient's chest.

We yelled for help and told Toby, the tech, to call a code. The patient was dying in front of us. The nurses got a set of vitals, and he had critically low blood pressure. We told them to call the surgeons. The residents arrived in a couple of minutes and assessed the situation. The chief told the residents to get the OR ready, but he was going to crack his chest here and now. They grabbed a thoracotomy tray from the ED and a few moments later, he sliced through the chest, and blood came gushing out. The patient's heart stopped beating, and they placed shock paddles directly on his heart and yelled "Clear!" They shocked his heart back into action, and then they whisked him off to the OR.

The amount of blood on the table, on the surgical drapes, and on the ground was unbelievable, but after the cleaning crew came, the room was ready to go for the next patient just twenty minutes later.

I found out later that day that the surgeons were unable to fix his aorta, and, despite their best efforts, he died in the OR.

24

THIRD RAIL

My GIRLFRIEND AND I were coming back to the city from spending a weekend in Connecticut. As my parents live there, I always had a place to stay when I needed to get away from the city. Although I had a car, it was easier to take the subway to Manhattan and jump on a train to Connecticut. I could use the ride time to catch up on sleep.

I got back to the city at about 7:00 p.m. after a nice weekend in the country. We hopped on the subway with our backpacks. However, just a few stops later, the train came to an abrupt stop. I was half-asleep, and didn't understand the announcement that came over the notoriously muffled and incomprehensible speaker. But it seemed that all the passengers were leaving our car. I stuck my head out the door and saw that most of the passengers were exiting the train and heading away from the platform.

We grabbed our bags and left the subway car. I noticed a subway worker standing next to our car as we walked out. He was looking under the car at the tracks. Reflexively, I looked down where he was looking, and saw a body sprawled out under the subway car. I looked at my girlfriend and then at the subway worker. I decided that as a doctor, I had an obligation to see if I could help. All kinds of thoughts went whizzing through my mind.

"Call 911," I barked at the worker.

I started to climb down from the platform onto the tracks.

"Watch out for the third rail," the worker warned me as he got out his radio.

"Third rail?" I asked.

"Yeah, fifteen hundred volts," he informed me.

"Which one?" I asked.

"Not sure," he said.

"Okay…" I stopped myself from going any further. I lay prone on the platform and tried to get a good look at the victim.

"Jumper," he said into the radio.

I could see the victim's legs, and they weren't moving. There was blood on his shirt. I could see his chest, but I couldn't be certain he was breathing. I decided to wait for the EMTs, because one victim was enough. I looked down at the tracks. The third rail is the one that carries the electricity. It should be pretty obvious where it is, but I couldn't figure it out.

The EMTs arrived after about five minutes. I told them I was a doctor and was willing to help if they needed it. I told them what I knew and had seen.

They went down onto the tracks without hesitation and were able to secure his neck and place him on a backboard. They brought him up to the platform and asked me what I thought.

The top of his head was bashed in or missing. He was gurgling and he breathed at near-death frequency.

"Not good," I said, "but he's alive…for the moment. We should secure his airway. Do you guys have a tube?"

The EMTs opened their case and placed a breathing tube as best they could under the circumstances. They whisked him away. A police officer took down my name and information. It felt weird.

I hadn't really helped, but I think my presence there made the EMTs feel a little more comfortable.

I grabbed my backpack and took another train home. A few days later, an officer called me to finish taking a statement and thanked me for helping out.

At the end of the conversation, I asked him, "By the way, how did he do?"

"Oh...he was DOA," he said nonchalantly. "Good thing you didn't go down onto the tracks. Hate to have two."

(Incidentally, the next day was busier at the County than usual. It was the day when the World Trade Center was attacked for the first time. A bomb exploded in the parking garage. Although almost forgotten because of the more serious events that followed, this attack occurred in 1993, eight years before the towers were destroyed on September 11, 2001. Patients were transported to hospitals all over the city, including Kings County Hospital. Only six people died in the attack, but over one thousand were injured.)

25

THE BIGGER THEY ARE

K INGS COUNTY HOSPITAL had not really changed that much since the days of Walter Reed. Patients who were to be evaluated for medical problems were placed in either the Male Room or the Female Room. These were large open rooms often filled with patients on stretchers. There were no curtains or privacy screens between the patients.[16] My patient was Mr. Francois. I called out his name and he answered. He was two rows back, and I had to squeeze past a gurney to get to him.

The chart said he was six feet four inches tall and weighed 275 pounds—a very large man. I crawled in between the stretchers, the stethoscope in my lab coat pocket catching on everything. I had a few pens in my pocket as well as a small notebook containing preprinted cards to write down patients' data in shorthand. I also kept an assortment of blood tubes, needles, gloves, and rubber tubing in my pockets for drawing blood. Most of my stuff landed on the ground when I hung up my stethoscope.

I picked up the fallen detritus and introduced myself to Mr. Francois. He had a heavy Caribbean accent, the rhythmic singsong

16 Lisa Belkin, "Accreditation Peril Faced by Kings County Hospital," *New York Times*, January 30, 1992.

of such an islander. He seemed very frightened, which seemed to contest with his large stature. He told me he had had a cough for a month and was worried. He looked so healthy and strong, I couldn't imagine what could have cut him down.

I reviewed his ER chart and noted he didn't have a fever. His blood pressure was normal. They had taken a chest X-ray, which was written on the X-ray jacket as "Negative for pneumonia. Nodule?"

After interviewing him and writing an admission note, I went to hunt down his X-ray.

The X-rays were taken across the hall, placed in large manila envelopes, and brought over in a bin to the radiology residents' room—the box. The resident would dictate a report into a tape recorder / Dictaphone and scribble a few words on the envelope. Then the resident would put the jacket into the back of the bin. The bin would be brought back to the file room later, and if the patient had an X-ray jacket, the new films would be placed in the jacket.

I flirted with the file-room clerk, and between the two of us, I was able to find Mr. Francois's films and signed them out. I brought them over to the radiologist and asked him to review the films with me. He said there was no pneumonia, but he was concerned about a few shadows he thought might be nodules. Honestly, I couldn't see them, but I nodded my head. He thought a CT scan might be helpful. I asked him what he thought the nodules were.

"Not certain...could be TB," he said.

That made sense to me. We saw a lot of TB, and he had a cough and was from Haiti. He might also be HIV positive. It seemed it was all coming together. I decided to place a TB skin test on his left wrist and a control on his right. The TB skin test will turn positive in about forty-eight hours if the patient has been exposed to TB. The control was used because if his immune system were compromised (i.e., if he had AIDS), the control would be negative, and the TB test could also be negative... even if he had TB.

With 80 percent of my patients having HIV or AIDS, it was imperative to test for TB, but without the control solution, the results of the skin test could be meaningless. At Kings County Hospital, we always had the TB test solution, which I could get at any nursing station, but we rarely had the control solution. However, the hospital across the street, SUNY Downstate, had the control solution. Since I worked on both sides of the street, I managed to keep a supply of the control solution in my lab coat for situations like this. I felt like Radar from *M*A*S*H*. That was the way the world was then.

Mr. François arrived on A71. It was a huge coincidence, but his nurse happened to be his ex-wife. She told me they had been divorced for five years. It didn't seem to faze either one of them. Her presence did not seem to alleviate his fears. He told me he thought he was going to die. I reassured him we would soon figure out what the problem was.

I presented Mr. Francois to my resident that evening and to the attending on rounds the next morning, and we made a plan. My attending was a pulmonologist and wanted us to do a pleural biopsy. He thought we might have a better chance of making the diagnosis that way, and he thought his fellow needed the practice. They would do that this morning because they were here. We would also order a CT scan and see what that showed and await the results of the TB and control skin tests. *We should have this worked out in forty-eight hours and I'll discharge him,* I thought.

After we performed the biopsy, the radiology resident said they had time to do his CT scan that afternoon. Bonus—he wasn't scheduled until the next day! He said, if I would bring him down right away, we could get it done that day.

It turned out I had a history with this resident's med school roommate. His girlfriend Hanna broke up with him to be with me, but I already had a girlfriend back home in Connecticut. It was during our first year of medical school and I wasn't certain if it was going to work out with the girl back home. Hanna and I had flirted during class, and I had given her a rose for Valentine's Day. Her soon-to-be ex discovered the rose, and she told him about me. However, I decided that I wasn't interested in more than flirting. As it turned out, one of my friends had a huge crush on her, and they ultimately got married.

I got a wheelchair and helped Mr. Francois sit. He barely fit in the chair. I pushed the chair down the hallway and onto the elevator. We got off the elevator on the second floor, and I pushed him down the long hallway between A and B Buildings. The light streamed in from the window, creating long shadows, and every few feet, the sunlight blinded me temporarily. I trudged on to the CT scanner room.

The tech opened the door for us and got Mr. Francois onto the CT table. I went into the control booth and chatted with the resident. I couldn't help but reflect on what had happened with his old roommate. It felt awkward.

The tech started the scan and the slices started coming up on the screen. The radiology resident and I reviewed the images as they came up. Even though I was just a medical student, I could tell it was bad, really bad. On every slice, there were white balls—masses. It seemed unreal to me. I looked to the resident, and he said it was metastatic disease. He even had one large mass that was attached to his pericardium (the sac around the heart).

"We could biopsy one," the resident said, "but it probably won't matter."

I got the wheelchair and helped Mr. Francois off the CT table. He asked me how it looked.

I couldn't help myself. I said, "Not good."

He didn't say anything. He just got back into the wheelchair. I could swear he'd lost fifty pounds since I brought him down. The mountain of a man no longer felt that way to me. I pushed him back to the elevator in silence. The sun was behind us now, and the shadows were even longer in the hallway. Neither of us wanted to talk. I was in shock, and his fears were confirmed.

A few days later, Mr. Francois started to collect fluid in his lungs and more ominously, fluid around his heart. He was getting sicker and frailer. The fluid around his heart was caused by one of the tumors invading his pericardium, (the thick sac around the heart) which responds by creating fluid. The fluid restricts the normal motion of the heart, and it can't pump well. He was dying in front of me. I think he knew when he came into the ED that this was happening; that was why he was so scared. I had thought it was just early TB.

That night, his heart was struggling so much that they moved him into the ICU. The cardiothoracic surgeons took him to the OR and created a pericardial window (a hole in the pericardium) to drain the fluid away from his heart so it could pump more effectively. However, during the surgery they discovered even worse news, that the tumors were not only invading his pericardium, they were also invading his heart muscle itself.

I saw Mr. Francois one more time on rounds before he died in the ICU. He had lost even more weight and looked frailer than ever.

26

OVER MY DEAD BODY!

"OVER MY DEAD body!" I screamed at my senior resident, Eddy. I was trying to discharge one of my patients, who had come into the hospital four days earlier with bronchopneumonia. She was eighty-two years old and lived independently. Her daughter had gone over to her apartment and had observed her coughing and took her temperature. She had a fever of 101°F. Her daughter insisted on bringing her mother to the hospital. The mother responded well to the antibiotics and was ready to be discharged. On rounds, I informed Eddy I was arranging for her daughter to pick her up at 10:00 a.m.

Eddy had finished his internship and was now one of the senior residents. I was still a lowly intern. Eddy's accent had worn off considerably over the past two years. When I met him, he was drowning with patients on his service. Now, he was the senior resident, in charge of four interns. Now, he was *my* senior resident, and he had a serious chip on his shoulder. He wanted the four of us interns to share in the pain and frustration he had when he was an intern. He seemed to arbitrarily raise the bar for our discharges, ostensibly to do the best thing for the patients.

Eddy said something to me that infuriated me. It sent me into such a rage that I was going to hit him—hard. He was my height and about my weight, but he didn't work out, and I spent most of my free time in the dojo.

What he told me was, "No patient will be discharged with a hematocrit of less than thirty-five. Give them two units of blood before they leave the hospital and they will feel much better."

I couldn't believe what he was saying. Many patients with chronic diseases have low hematocrits, and there are countless other reasons why patients might have a low hematocrit. But transfusing patients just to correct a number is preposterous and dangerous.

At that time, the blood supply was not tested for many things that are standard today such as HIV and hepatitis C (back then it was known as hepatitis non A–non B). I was not about to give an eighty-two-year-old woman who came in for simple pneumonia and had a HCT of 32 an HIV infection just so, according to Eddy, she would feel a little better. I would rather knock his head off and get kicked out of the program than do something as wanton and idiotic as he proposed.

Consider that Arthur Ashe, the number-one tennis player in the world in 1968, developed premature significant coronary artery disease. He had bypass surgery in 1979. He was trying to make a comeback, but suffered chest pain again, and underwent a second bypass surgery in New York. Most people believe that during his second bypass procedure in 1983 he received a tainted blood transfusion and became infected with the HIV virus. He died of complications from AIDS-related pneumonia in 1993.[17] Before his death, he created the Arthur Ashe Institute for Urban Health,[18] which aims to improve community health initiatives for minorities. He chose to establish the Institute in partnership with Downstate because it was in the heart of Brooklyn, treating patients from

17 http://www.biography.com/people/arthur-ashe-9190544

18 http://www.arthurasheinstitute.org/arthurashe/home/

a multitude of different ethnicities and cultures. The Institute opened in 1992, the year of my graduation from Downstate.

I was not going to allow my little old lady patient to die of AIDS like Arthur Ashe. She had recovered nicely from pneumonia. I was not certain why her hematocrit was low, but it could be addressed as an outpatient by her internist. Some acutely sick patients drop their hematocrit based on the temporary suppression of the synthesis of blood in the bone marrow secondary to the illness. She could be anemic from blood loss due to an occult GI malignancy or a host of other issues. None of these would require her to stay an extra minute in the hospital at this time.

I'm sure Eddy felt he was right because he probably had learned that strategy from someone, but I'd be damned if I was going to put my patient in harm's way for someone else's irrational beliefs. *Primum non nocere* ("First do no harm," part of the Hippocratic Oath). I think he realized he was being unreasonable, and ultimately, he let me discharge her as long as I alerted her primary care physician to the fact that she was anemic.

27

CODE RED

"CODE RED A71! Code Red A71!"

We were in the middle of rounds on A11.

"Shit! Code Red? A71?" I looked at my resident and he gave me a nod of recognition.

"That's us," I said, steeling myself for something really bad.

We broke into a run and headed toward the nearest staircase. We bolted up the stairs, taking them two at time. Most of us were in pretty good shape because we ran up and down eight flights of stairs routinely many times a day. We had patients scattered from the eighth floor of A Building (A71 and A72) down to the second floor (A11 and A12).

Normally, as part of the medical code team, we get called for Code Blue, which is when a patient is in respiratory distress and dying. We run from wherever we are and usually get to the patient's bed, and get a report from whoever witnessed the event as we gather other information before making an assessment. The majority of the time, the patient's airway will need to be stabilized, and ultimately an endotracheal tube will be placed down the trachea and the patient will be placed on a ventilator. The patient may be having a heart attack or their heart was going into an abnormal rhythm, in which case we try to resuscitate them using ACLS (advanced cardiovascular life support), protocols with drugs, and/or shocking the heart.

I was pretty comfortable in this situation. It was basically cookbook stuff. The hardest part was catching my breath and getting my emotions under control. The first thing I would tell myself was, "It isn't happening to me. I'm not the one dying." This phrase seemed to help me focus on the tasks at hand and remove the fear and anxiety. It allowed me to do my job methodically and to think clearly, especially if I knew the patient well and had created a bond with them. It was still not me who was in trouble. My job was to stay calm and try to help them get through this. The problem is, some residents freak out and start barking orders at everyone. I found this strategy to be counterproductive. The staff stop thinking about doing their job and start thinking about how to avoid getting yelled at.

Code Red means someone is bleeding to death, very unusual on the medical wards. I felt ill-prepared for this and had a sinking feeling in my chest as we ran down the hallway to the multi-patient room where a crowd of staff was forming.

Crap! When we entered the room, I saw it was my patient who was in distress. Mr. Hilaire had been my patient for two weeks. He was a thirty-four-year-old Haitian man with AIDS. He had spent the past couple of months in the County being treated for active TB. First he was in the TB isolation ward on A32 for four weeks, and then he was transferred to the regular wards to finish his course of antibiotics before, hopefully, his family would take him home.

Although he was skinny, five feet nine inches tall and 135 pounds, he otherwise looked and acted totally healthy. He walked around the ward like he owned it: sometimes he would join us on rounds when we were on his floor. He had a chessboard and we had an ongoing game. He even had me paged once to ask me what my next move was.

Mr. Hilaire was sitting up in his bed. His eyes met mine when I burst into the room, and I could see the fear that emanated from them. He was coughing up blood—bright-red blood. Blood that was coming from an artery in his chest. Blood that we were not going to be able to stop anytime soon. He coughed again and blood came shooting out across the bed. He looked at me, pleading for me to save his life.

My resident and I started barking out orders to get more help. We put on our gowns, goggles, and gloves. We opened the crash cart (a cart that contains medications and equipment used in emergencies). He didn't even have an IV! His heart stopped about ten minutes in. We tried everything we could to revive his heart, but were unsuccessful. He passed out a few moments later. We worked on him for the next thirty minutes. We placed an endotracheal tube, sent someone for blood, placed an IV, and then placed a central venous catheter. A team of surgeons came in during the middle of all this. Blood was everywhere. They stared at us for a few minutes and then told us to give them a call if we got him stabilized, knowing full well there was no chance of that.

I heard one of them mumble, "Let's get out of the Killing Fields while we still can."

After we removed our surgical gowns, masks, and gloves, and left the gory man who once was my patient, my resident and I spoke to each other. "What do you think happened to him?" the resident asked.

Interesting question. During that whole episode, I had not even asked myself why he was bleeding to death. I was so focused on just trying to get control of the situation, I never stopped to think about why it was happening.

I felt stupid for not even having given it a thought and strained to recall everything I knew about him. I thought he was healthy and going home soon. *What had I missed?* I felt a pang of fear that his death was somehow my fault. I started to panic. I considered what I knew about him. Haitian male, HIV positive, TB. That was it.

My resident saw I was struggling and bailed me out.

"His TB eroded from the lung into a major artery, maybe a bronchial artery or even the aorta," he said. "I've seen it back home in Pakistan a couple of times. Nasty way to die. Comes on suddenly and there's nothing we can do."

Wow! I knew people died of TB, but I had never experienced anything like that.

To this day, I can still see his eyes, pleading for me to do something to save him.

28

HOLE IN THE GROUND

KINGS COUNTY HOSPITAL is a very old hospital. Most of the structures were built in the 1930s, so the infrastructure was out of date. The floor plan was from a long-gone era. The AIDS epidemic was ravaging the poor black communities living in Brooklyn and the thousand-bed hospital didn't seem to be big enough. The city decided to construct a new hospital on the campus of the County in 1984.

The plan was to build a new twelve-hundred-bed hospital next to the original structure, directly across the street from Downstate Hospital. To do this, several of the old buildings needed to be demolished. The existing infrastructure, conduits, wires, and sewer lines all needed to be moved to accommodate a new building in the middle of the existing city campus. The city promised to allocate contracts for the project to minority and women subcontractors to try to revitalize an area of Brooklyn that had slid into poverty. Hopes were high.

However, the project was very complex, and, like many large and politically charged projects, it imploded. A few buildings were demolished, and the dirt left behind was smoothed into parking lots. A small staff cafeteria, which was sorely needed because there was no cafeteria at the County, was constructed in one of the ancillary buildings. That needs repeating: at a thousand-bed hospital there was no place to eat in the building except for a couple of vending machines. The residents sometimes worked twenty-four-hour or thirty-six-hour shifts! I had heard of residents ordering extra food for their patients so they could co-opt it for themselves: for example, ordering a regular diet for a patient who was already getting tube feeds or IV nutrition. The surrounding neighborhood was blighted and the only place to get any food was a small Caribbean pastry and coffee shop across the street.

It was asserted that the delays in building the new County cost $100,000 a day. After years of mismanagement costing the city over $100 million, the project was shut down. According to Luis A. Miranda Jr., the chairman of New York's Health and Hospitals Corporation, "After having spent $119 million to date, we have only an administrative building, a food service building, a couple of holes in the ground, a few parking lots and some pictures of past mayors with hard hats claiming they have fulfilled a promise."[19] Mayor Rudolph Giuliani shut the project down in 1994.

---

19 David Firestone, "New York Hospitals Chief Calls Brooklyn Plan a Giant Failure," *New York Times*, February 11, 1994.

29

DEAD HEROES

W E WERE FORTUNATE enough to add a new, young superstar surgeon to our staff in 1994. Dr. Warren Wetzel was chief of trauma surgery at Jacobi Medical Center in the Bronx from 1986 until 1994. He came to Downstate and Kings County Hospital at the age of forty-five and immediately became one of the most loved attending surgeons among the residents. Even though he was a big-time surgeon, he seemed approachable and likeable. He was one of those energetic go-getter types and always had a good attitude.

During rounds one day, one of the residents pointed out to him that he could have approached the situation differently, and the patient probably would have benefited.

Dr. Wetzel nodded his head and said, "Learn something new every day."

Dr. Sal Sclafani, the head of interventional radiology at the County and a leader in the field of interventional radiology and trauma, was one of Warren's new friends. He had been stricken with severe flank pain. A CT scan performed on him revealed an obstructing stone in his ureter. A few weeks later, Dr. Wetzel also had flank pain and he got a CT scan as well. Unfortunately, it uncovered the fact that he had a mass in his pelvis and had metastases to the lymph nodes in his abdomen and pelvis. He was diagnosed with an aggressive form of prostate cancer. He underwent cancer therapy, and I remember him stopping by one day after trauma rounds to hop on the CT scanner to get follow-up scans. He asked me to go over the scans with him. I told him that things looked about the same as before.

He died tragically in March of 1996, at the age of forty-seven, only two short years after coming to the County.[20]

We were also fortunate to have another surgeon, Dr. Herrera, who specialized in liver cancer, join the staff. He was in his fifties. He wanted to treat cancers of the liver aggressively, initially by giving chemotherapy directly to the liver by placing a catheter in the hepatic artery. This was a technically difficult procedure, snaking the catheter out into the small arteries that directly feed the tumor. It took time, patience, and skill to get the catheter to follow the curves of the hepatic artery to only deliver the medications to the cancerous tissue. Then we would hook up a device to deliver the chemotherapy overnight into the tumor. Over the next few weeks, we would monitor the patient with CT scans. If the tumor regressed, Dr. Herrera would try to remove the cancer or the diseased portion of the liver.

We were excited to be involved in this complex and innovative care. We had done the procedure on five patients, and it seemed like the program was taking off. Unfortunately, while on vacation, Dr. Herrera had a heart attack and died unexpectedly. The new treatment program died with him.

---

20 "Dr. Warren Wetzel, Trauma Surgeon, 47," *New York Times*, March 29, 1996.

30

MY BETROTHED

ALL RADIOLOGY RESIDENTS finish their residency by taking the
board exam in Louisville, Kentucky, at the beginning of June.
We study for four years, and it culminates in a hotel in Kentucky
where cases are shown in hotel rooms and the applicant is grilled
by an attending for thirty minutes. At the sound of a bell, the resident leaves that session and moves on to the next hotel room on
their list and more grilling.

I had studied hard and felt relieved when it was over. During
my training, we had a case conference every day at lunch. A different attending would present cases every day and grill the residents
to get them prepared for the oral boards. I realized early on in my
training that the attendings would usually start with a softball case
and then present progressively harder cases. Most of the residents
tried to avoid getting called. I decided I was going to volunteer
to be first every day, something I did almost without fail for four
years. I would take my case, answer questions, and then sit down
and eat my lunch in peace.

After all that practice, I felt pretty confident I had passed my
boards. I couldn't wait to celebrate! In a few short weeks, my stint
in New York would come to an end—finally! My fiancée, Chi-Na,

had convinced me that there was life beyond the Hudson River and I expanded my search for fellowships outside of New York. I had been accepted at a very prestigious neuroradiology fellowship at the Barrow Neurological Institute in Phoenix, Arizona. I couldn't believe the contrast between the County and the Barrow when I went there for my interview. I was ready to turn down all other job offers on the spot when I looked out the window. There were beautiful red-rock mountains in the Sonoran Desert in the vista from the hospital! The hospital was clean and ultramodern. There were three MRI scanners in the hospital! We converted to filmless imaging during my year at the Barrow. There were IV teams, blood-draw teams, transporters, monitors, computers, and even a cafeteria for the staff and patients.

I was looking forward to moving to Phoenix, even though Chi-Na and I would be apart. We went out to fancy restaurants in Brooklyn Heights and in Park Slope over the next few days celebrating my new job. We packed up Chi-Na's stuff and moved her into an apartment in Far Rockaway. I had arranged for a mover to pick up my stuff and started to pack my apartment into boxes.

The evening before the movers came, I went for a last ten-mile run with my best friend, Mitch. I started to have belly cramps during the last mile. When I got back to my apartment, the diarrhea started. I was sweating like crazy. I took a shower and got back to packing. Chi-Na had fallen asleep. The next morning Chi-Na went off to work in the ED at the County. I was feverish and weak and couldn't get out of bed. I had been sick like this a couple of times before in my life. The first time was when I was a freshman in college and contracted salmonella (typhoid fever). The second time was when I contracted traveler's diarrhea in Kathmandu during my internship. I continued to have diarrhea and continued to get weaker. I tried to pack up the rest of my stuff, but could barely get out of bed.

The movers came and saw they could take advantage of me. They offered to finish packing my stuff for me, but at an exorbitant price. I was in no position to argue with them, since I did not have the energy, and agreed to pay them my first two months' salary.

I called Chi-Na, and she thought I was faking it, that I just didn't want to pack or move and was being lazy. I told her I really was very sick, and she said I should come to the ED. I wasn't certain I was strong enough to even drive, but I decided to chance it. I felt so incredibly weak! When I got to the ED, Chi-Na placed me on a stretcher in the trauma bay. She hooked me up to monitors and registered my heart rate at eighty-eight beats per minute. Her attendings scoffed at me and said that was normal. Chi-Na realized I was in trouble, because although eighty-eight beats per minute is only slightly fast for most people, my resting heart rate was usually forty-four beats per minute. The equivalent heart rate for someone with a normal baseline of 70 beats per minute would be over 140 beats per minute. I was supposedly at rest, but my heart was working twice as hard as it should. Chi-Na put in a large-bore IV and started administering IV fluids. I started to feel better after an hour, but the diarrhea continued.

At the end of her shift and after several bags of IV fluids, she drove me back to her apartment because I no longer had a bed in my apartment—or anything in my apartment, for that matter. Unfortunately, we had not had time to set up her bed yet either, and we slept on the floor that night. Every hour or so, I would go to the bathroom and have diarrhea. By morning, the effects of the IV fluids had worn off, and I told her I thought I was going to die if I didn't get to a "real" hospital.

We drove to Connecticut and met my parents in their local hospital ER. They started IV fluids and took stool samples. They found *Campylobacter jejuni* in my stool and started me on antibiotics. They let me go to my parents' home with an IV in my arm and plenty of bags of fluid to keep myself hydrated. They gave me a prescription for antibiotics that we could fill at any pharmacy.

I started to feel better after receiving the IV fluids and initial antibiotics. However, I was exhausted and lay on my parents' couch. The next day, Chi-Na and my mom set out to pick up my antibiotics and do some shopping. They returned several hours later chatting about their shopping and the various types of jewelry cleaners. They walked into my room, noticed me still lying prostrate, looked at each other, and realized they had forgotten to pick up the antibiotics. My younger sister Danae realized what they had done, and was speechless. She was about to yell at my mom and future wife. Instead, we all burst out laughing hysterically.

As with all of my other adventures I had while I was at the County, I survived. I got my antibiotics and cleared the infection. I got well enough to get on an airplane a few days later than I had initially planned. I left for the next phase of my medical education in Phoenix, Arizona—ending my time at the County, for better and for worse.

Made in the USA
San Bernardino, CA
02 April 2015